MW00469417

F🥚🥚D
INTOLERANCE
What
it is
&
how to
cope
with it

F🥚🥚D
INTOLERANCE

What it is & how to cope with it

by ROBERT BUIST PhD

PRISM ALPHA

FOOD INTOLERANCE
What it is and how to cope with it

Copyright © 1984 Robert Buist

Published in Great Britain in 1984 by
Prism Press.
Marketed by Prism Alpha Ltd,
          Half Moon St.,
          Sherborne, Dorset DT9 3LN UK
and in the USA by Prism Alpha
          PO Box 778
          San Leandro
          CA 94577 USA

Originally published in Australia
by Harper & Row (Australasia) Pty Ltd.

ISBN 0 907061 68 0

First edition
Designed by Judy Hungerford
Edited by Kate Geoghegan Campbell
Printed and typeset at The Dominion Press-Hedges & Bell, Maryborough. Victoria 3465

NOTE:

SPECIAL DIET PLANS AND RECIPES FREE OF:

Wheat (other gluten containing foods have been strictly limited)

Dairy products (including milk, cheese, butter, cream, yogurt, lactose, powdered milk)

Yeast — moulds

Malt

Coffee

Tea

Sugar

Food additives

Chemicals

Foods are *rotated* in the diet plans to decrease *quantity* and *frequency* of consumption while increasing nutrient density.

Where possible, international equivalents are given for vegetables, fruits, grains and measurements. For example, paw paw/papaya, eggplant/aubergine, jelly/gelatin.

Everybody would like to know the cause of food intolerance but at the moment we just don't have a simple answer.

CONTENTS

CHAPTER 9

COPING WITH CHILDREN

ACKNOWLEDGEMENTS

The concept for this book arose primarily from a fairly standard question asked by a great majority of my patients with food hypersensitivities. It went something like this: 'Where can we get a recipe book that completely eliminates yeast, wheat and dairy products and is based on seasonal foods (recipes for different seasons) and also explains the do's and dont's of food intolerance in the form of a simple easy to follow program that can be carried out at home.' As I knew of no such book I was further urged to write one. This also gave me the opportunity to enlarge on some of my own clinical experiences which were sometimes at variance with other published approaches to food intolerance. It also enabled me to elaborate on the key factors involved in maximising patient compliance, the major factor in any new lifestyle program.

So the initial impetus and thanks goes to my patients who encouraged me to save at least half of the time involved in a consultation by writing down my instructions in the form of a book rather than my usual illegible scrawls.

With the continuing and indispensible help of Wendy, my wife, in diet design, food substitutions and preparation—the final book took shape.

I would especially like to thank Marj Allnutt for her untiring interest and support, Alwyn Simms, Jarni Boucher, Julie Allen, Pam Low, Lindy Kingsmill and Lynette Morgan for their ideas and contributions of tested recipes and the numerous members of the Sensitivity Awareness Organisation (SAO) for their encouragement and helpful discussions.

INTRODUCTION

Education and a little common sense tells most people that fresh or unprocessed whole foods must be the most suitable for the promotion of health. Numerous books have highlighted the health problems associated with an excessive consumption of sugar, salt, fat, refined carbohydrates, coffee, alcohol and tobacco. However important these findings may be, they do not mention that there may also be inherent dangers in eating totally nutritious foodstuffs. It has come as a shock to many people to learn that food intolerances are associated with such disorders as asthma, arthritis, scleraderma, multiple sclerosis, lupus erythematosus, Crohns disease, irritable bowel syndrome, skin complaints and even mental health problems such as schizophrenia, depression and agoraphobia. These food intolerances are not associated with some rare or exotic delicacies from distant shores, but rather to our most common daily foods which are frequently eaten. Some people decide to get rid of junk food and sugar from their diet and eat only whole unprocessed foods because of acute or chronic health problems only to find that their condition continues to deteriorate. In numerous cases the reason for this deterioration is an undetected food intolerance. Fortunately not everyone reacts in this way, but for those who do it can be the blight of their life.

Foods can have an adverse effect in many ways. Some are inadequately digested in the intestines because of a missing enzyme as demonstrated in lactose intolerance. For others there is a genetic susceptibility involving abnormal or missing intestinal enzymes as in gluten intolerance (coeliac disease). Inflammatory bowel conditions like irritable colon and Crohn's disease have now been linked with various food sensitivities. Partially digested proteins from foods such as wheat and milk can be absorbed systemically and cause migraines, others act on the brain in a similar fashion to morphine-like hormones. Such peptides are called exorphins and appear to be involved in some mental disorders, notably schizophrenia.

Other food peptides act as antigens and induce the body to make antibodies which subsequently form immune complexes which can cause inflammation and degeneration in the joints, bones and soft tissues. This is the case in rheumatoid arthritis and the collagen diseases and also in other so-called auto-immune disorders. Such reactions can be immediate hypersensitivity reactions (IgE mediated) as in hay fever, asthma, eczema or delayed allergic reactions involving other immunoglobulins Ig M, A, D, G. Some do not involve the immune system at all and are more related to changes in fatty acid metabolism and substances called prostaglandins. Reactive foods may also be those containing salicylates, phenols, preservatives, colourings or naturally occurring toxic substances which have been known to precipitate hyperactivity, aggressive behaviour, lack of concentration and short attention span. Toxic mineral contaminants in foods including lead, mercury, cadmium may effect learning, balance, co-ordination and fine motor movements. All of these food related hypersensitivity reactions result in adverse physiological changes in the body and encompass a much wider area than normally confined to the field of food allergy.

In this book I have mainly elaborated on the immunologically based reactions, but this has been for illustrative purposes only. While we are concerned about all types of food related hypersensitivity reactions we will be mainly focusing on the patient with multiple food sensitivities which seem to vary from day to day and which arise largely because of the consumption of an increased quantity of specific foods and with an increased frequency of consumption.

The two major foods which fit this category in Australia are products derived from cow's milk and wheat. Many are sensitised to these two food categories as infants and perhaps even in utero, while others suddenly become sensitised in later life after some stressful event in their lives suddenly precipitates all kinds of sensitivities to not only foods, but also to house dust, chemicals, pollen, moulds and any number of previously innocuous substances.

Yeast-containing-foods including vegemite, brewers yeast, torula yeast, breads, beer and wines have also been eliminated from the recipes in this book largely because of the work of C. Orian Truss,[60] a medical practitioner from Birmingham, Alabama, who showed that chronic infection with Candida albicans may also be a major factor in the expression of food intolerance in the person with suboptimal immunological responses.

The easiest and most constructive way of finding and eliminating such food sensitivities is to completely remove the most common troublemakers from the daily diet for a fixed period of time while, at the same time, rotating the remaining foods in moderate quantities so that a completely different selection of foods is eaten each day. With the specific food 'stressors' either removed completely or consumed less frequently the body has a chance of recovering and most foods can then be reintroduced, but with a careful eye on quantity and frequency of consumption.

Unfortunately this is not the end of the story. The expression of the most common types of food intolerance depends upon a multifactoral system of which the food itself constitutes only one part. The final allergic manifestations depend upon the following additional factors.

a Interaction of external environmental factors including moulds, yeasts, fungus, house dust, pollens, chemicals, viruses, bacteria, temperature, weather changes and so on.
b The emotional and mental state of the individual and associated body stress levels.
c The input of positive antistress factors such as aerobic exercise, nutrient intake, rest and active forms of mental relaxation.

Of particular relevance for this book is the emotional and mental state of the food intolerant individual and special emphasis is placed on this area. During the last century Sir William Osler, the father of modern medicine, said: 'The care of tuberculosis depends more on what the patient has in his head than what he has on his chest.' It is now quite clear that the way we perceive a stressful situation (rather than the actual stressful situation itself) is what strongly influences our state of health. Failure to cope with stress can reduce a person's ability to fight off illness by significantly impairing immunological responses. Strong emotional reactions can actually stimulate the course of a disease. Researchers at Mount Sinai Medical Centre in New York, Drs. Schliefer, Stein and Keller have recently shown that a family bereavement such as the death of a wife from breast cancer, will cause a sharp decline in the function of the husband's white blood cells several months before the death. Animal experiments have similarly demonstrated that cancers will grow faster in stressed animals. Animals kept in cramped 'high stress' housing conditions will secrete large levels of the adrenal hormone, corticosterone and exhibit a decline in white blood cells and thymus gland function (the master gland of the immune system) compared to animals housed in a 'low stress' environment.

The emotional and mental health of the food intolerant person is a key factor and has frequently given rise to snide accusations such as 'it's all in the mind' or 'it's purely psychological'. The psychosomatic component of asthma has always been recognised and we are beginning to realise the vast psychological implications for all forms of immunological based diseases and other stress related disorders.

When all these factors are recognised and appropriate dietary and lifestyle modifications undertaken, the reduction in total body stress burden results in the elimination of most cases of food intolerance.

CHAPTER 1

FOOD
INTOLERANCE

THE PROTEIN ATTACK

In normal health, the protein components in our foods are broken down by digestive enzymes (juices) in our body to yield amino acids. These are then absorbed through our gastrointestinal tract and either burned up to supply us with energy or recombined to form the particular protein that our body requires for making muscles, tissues, skin, enzymes etc.

Obviously, the proteins from eggs, chicken or beef cannot be incorporated directly into our own tissues but through the process of digestion we are able to break down 'foreign' egg or beef protein into its component parts (amino acids) and then recombine them as human proteins which have different sequences of amino acids. The human proteins have the same amino acid building blocks but are completely different from other animal proteins in nature.

So the digestive juices in our body break down all foreign proteins, preventing their direct absorption into the body. If some of these protein components actually enter the body we go on red alert and our immune system is brought into play in the same way that it comes to our rescue if a virus or bacteria gets into our system. That is, the body steps up its defense mechanism against invading foreign allergenic protein components in the same manner that it does against viruses and bacteria. It does this by calling into action certain white blood cells which travel through the blood stream (some are actually stationed in our tissues) and when they find one of these foreign proteins (be they from virus, bacteria or undigested food) they engulf them, digest them and destroy them. This is the job of our immune system, the great protector of our body from colds, flu and even cancer, arthritis and other chronic diseases. It is our second line of defense against invading undigested food substances, and is of great importance to the person with food allergies.

The first line of defence is our digestive system which works hand in hand with our immuno-defence system to protect the body from the onslaught of unwelcome guests. These may take the form of pollens, house mites, cat fur, dog skin, viruses, moulds, yeast, milk, egg, wheat protein and so on depending upon individual susceptibility.

In general our digestive juices and special digestive enzymes, which are stationed in the lining of our small intestines, are quite capable of screening out these foreign proteins. In fact proteins are not supposed to enter the body at all. However, in some susceptible individuals either one or both of these two protective mechanisms, the digestive system and the immune system, are malfunctional and this can lead to all the problems that we associated with food and environmental sensitivities.

Two obvious examples that spring to mind are lactose intolerance and coeliac disease. A lactose intolerant person, for example, does not have the required intestinal enzymes to digest lactose (the sugar found in milk). As a result of this malfunction of digestion the lactose sugar remains in the gut undigested and tends to draw water from the body into the intestines. At the same time intestinal bacteria cause the lactose to ferment. This generates lactic acid, other organic acids, carbon dioxide and hydrogen, resulting in bloating, flatulence, cramps and diarrhoea.

A person who cannot tolerate wheat products or other gluten containing foods has a similar problem called coeliac disease. These individuals have to maintain a diet free from wheat, rye, barley and oats because all of these foods contain a group of proteins called gluten which yield toxic fragments (peptides) which can injure the cells lining the small intestine. One theory suggests that this occurs because of an abnormal (either defective or deficient) enzyme in the intestinal cells which fails to digest the toxic peptide fragment. At any rate, the absorptive surfaces of the intestines become damaged, are flattened and atrophy. This subsequently gives rise to the malabsorption of fats, carbohydrate, protein, vitamins (especially the fat soluble ones) and minerals. If gluten is removed from the diet of people with this type of food sensitivity the intestinal lining can return to normal but they must stay away from all gluten containing foods.

The biggest problem associated with these types of disorders is the malabsorption of nutrients which retards adequate growth and predisposes the individual to various types of illness. In both of the above mentioned examples the food related problems occur at the level of the gut. However, food sensitivities do not stop here. We now have very good evidence that protein components of various foods can actually pass through the gut into the blood stream and can act on various tissues of the body to cause inflammation, redness, swelling and pain. Such reactions can occur in the joints (as in the case of rheumatoid arthritis), in the brain (many coeliac patients are also schizophrenics), in the nose, throat and lung (as in rhinitis, bronchitis and asthma).

When such protein fragments attack the brain they do not necessarily cause such an extreme reaction as schizophrenia, but they can be associated with behaviour modification such as depression, uncooperative behaviour, irritability, short attention span and hyperactivity. Indeed studies in the US have shown a high correlation between the ingestion of excessive amounts of dairy products and soft drinks and juvenile delinquency. Feingold observed that salicylates and other food additives induced behaviour changes. But he only scratched the surface by not recognising the behavioural changes elicited by various foods themselves.

It is often difficult to believe that good nutritious foods such as wholegrain wheat products, cow's milk and free range eggs may be responsible for abnormal behaviour patterns, not to mention chronic disorders such as arthritis and asthma. Nevertheless, the potential is there and susceptibilities vary from individual to individual.

The most critical time in the development of food intolerance stems from the period of foetal life in the uterus and during the first year or two as an infant. While food sensitivities appear to be handed down from parents to offspring (especially if both parents have allergies) it is most important for the mother to abstain from any foods to which she is allergic during her pregnancy and also during the breast-feeding period. This is because some of the toxic food fragments may pass through the placenta to the foetus from the mother's blood and during lactation food allergens may pass through the breast milk to the infant.

During the first three weeks of life (and frequently this time extends to six months) the infant's intestines will let large protein molecules into the body. This is because the mother's milk contains special proteins called immunoglobulins which are supposed to penetrate the infant's intestines and pass into the blood stream to prime the newborn's immune system. One of these immunoglobulins called IgA actually binds to the infant's intestinal tract and acts as a screening agent for all foreign proteins. This is the prime function of the immunoglobulins. They are most concentrated in the colostrum and protect the infant from infectious diseases, viruses, bacteria, etc. The main problem arises if, during this time, other foreign proteins get through the baby's intestinal lining as well as the welcome immunoglobulins. While these phenomena are minor factors for the breastfed baby whose mother is not trying to avoid food allergens or does not have food sensitivities, it is a major problem for potential food-sensitive infants who at birth are immediately placed on soy-based formulas, cow's milk or other fluids containing foreign proteins.

During this early period the infant's digestive system is immature, protective intestinal antibodies such as IgA are absent, and the generally increased permeability of the immature intestines makes the infant a prime candidate for the development of food allergies or subsequent maladaptive food reactions related to the penetration of food proteins or protein fragments into the body. For this reason exposure of the infant to any food besides breast milk should be delayed for as long as possible, at least for 6-7 months. After this period the baby's digestive tract has matured enough to handle certain foreign proteins. Leave eggs, wheat and dairy products till last on your food introduction program.

SCIENTIFIC EVIDENCE FOR FOOD INTOLERANCE

During the last few years extensive research has indicated that the ingestion of dairy products, gluten-containing foods and/or a number of other types of foods may give rise to a great variety of different clinical disorders. These include chronic eczema, hay fever, bronchitis, asthma, and other respiratory disorders; diarrhoea, rheumatoid arthritis, schizophrenia, depression, migraines, and many others. Lets examine some of the evidence for the food related clinical disorders.

Several animal studies have demonstrated that blood proteins and other large molecular weight substances can gain entry to the bloodstream by bypassing the usual screening systems.[1] During the first week of life, rabbits rapidly absorb radioactive bovine serum albumin (BSA), a common protein found in cow's milk.[2] By the second and third weeks, however, the absorption stops. A 1977 report in the Lancet showed that there is also good evidence that neonatal exposure to cow proteins may be associated with the later development of childhood eczema and asthma.[3] The absorption of large molecular weight polymers similar in size to cow protein has also been demonstrated in eczema patients by researchers from Guy's Hospital Medical School, London.[4]

In one study involving 46 Indonesian children under the age of two who had diarrhoea, 33 had abnormal lining of the small intestine, and 20 of these infants showed improvement when cow's milk was withdrawn from the diet.[5] Investigators at the Royal Children's Hospital, Parkville, Victoria, Australia have found increases in specific serum antibodies in 54 children allergic to cow's milk protein.[6] Even gastrointestinal bleeding has been induced by cow's milk in certain children,[7] and there is one report of a child who developed urticaria and respiratory distress after the application of an ointment containing casein, the major protein derived from cow's milk.[8]

There is now increasing evidence that many of our chronic degenerative diseases such as rheumatoid arthritis may have their origin in adverse food reactions occurring during the postnatal period, when the immature intestinal tract has failed to screen out foreign proteins or peptides. This could continue through the early childhood period, and well into adolescence and adulthood. Adults also show immune responses after oral exposure to the cow protein called bovine serum albumin.[9]

The possible role of such allergenic macromolecules (toxic food fragments) in clinical disorders is well illustrated by the case of a 38-year-old woman with an 11-year history of degenerative rheumatoid arthritis, who became symptom free shortly after removing all dairy products from her diet[10] – intense synovitis and morning stiffness diminished and eventually disappeared. Marked improvements were also found in grip strength, ability to move joints and pain levels. There was an immediate reduction in her systemic inflammation and the complete disappearance of milk protein-antibody complexes in her blood stream. When she was re-exposed to cheese and milk after a 10-month symptom free period their was a 'pronounced deterioration of the patient's arthritis' within 24 hours, with an increase in morning stiffness and a decrease in grip strength. Laboratory findings at this time revealed deterioration in all parameters measured and the woman's immune system started producing antibodies again to combat the milk and cheese protein.

A relationship between the ingestion of dairy products and various forms of thought disorders in susceptible individuals has recently been demonstrated by Dr W M Bowerman.[11] Following unsuccessful conventional treatment, five psychiatric patients (schizophrenics and depressives) were placed on a dairy-free diet. After four days without milk, butter or yoghurt, most of the mental symptoms of all five patients in this study subsided. These symptoms included agitation, hallucinations, poor memory, confusion, insomnia, headaches, depression, fatigue, amnesia, 'spacey periods', learning difficulties, fuzzy thinking and explosive temper outbursts. A return of symptoms was noted in one patient who began consuming skim milk after considerable craving periods. All symptoms cleared when skim milk was again eliminated from the diet.

Other researchers have shown that these food reactions are not confined to milk and beef (bovine) proteins. The gluten fraction of wheat has also been implicated on many occasions.

In a recent report from the Royal Society of Medicine, Swain and Unsworth[12] have shown that patients with dermatitis herpetiformis had gluten specific antibodies (antigliadin) in their blood which disappeared as soon as the patients commenced a strict gluten-free diet (gliadin is a major protein component in the gluten fraction of wheat). A similar reduction in elevated anti-gluten antibodies was demonstrated in the blood of untreated coeliac children after they commenced a gluten-free diet, and reappeared after subsequent re-exposure to gluten containing foods.

The immunological reaction of psychiatric patients to fractions of wheat gluten has been documented.[13] Several investigators have shown that schizophrenic patients deteriorate when wheat gluten is added to their diet[14,15]. Dr Dohan, a researcher who has observed a correlation between various psychiatric disorders and cereal grain intake, has observed that schizophrenia occurs more frequently than by chance in patients with coeliac disease[16,17,18] and hospital admissions and length of stay of schizophrenic patients is highly correlated with cereal grain consumption[19]. Another study has revealed that 54 per cent of a group of psychiatric patients have antibodies to cereal proteins, compared with 19 per cent of a control group.[20] In other words the immune system of many psychiatric patients has been mobilised to fight these foreign cereal proteins that have entered the body.

Many different foods, in fact, can be allergenic for certain people depending upon individual susceptibilities. Some patients complain of multiple symptoms in spite of no confirmed organic diagnoses. This was the case for 12 patients reported in The Practitioner in 1981,[21] who claimed relief of symptoms after taking specific food exclusion diets for between 3 and 30 months. After reintroducing the excluded foods into the diet, 10 out of the 12 demonstrated a return of their original symptoms.

Dr Jean Monro and co-workers from the National Hospital for Nervous Diseases, Queens Square, London, have recently shown that 23 out of 33 migraine sufferers (70 per cent) were allergic to certain foods and elimination of these foods gave almost complete relief of migraines within about two weeks.[22] Subsequent food challenges predictably reproduced the migraines and a good correlation was found between clinically suspected foods and the presence of specific antibodies in the blood against these foods.

More recently 93 per cent of children aged 3-16 years suffering from severe and frequent migraine attacks were found to recover when placed on an oligoantigenic diet.[61] An oligoantigenic diet consists basically of eating only one of the main food types each day for 3-4 weeks — notably one meat (lamb or chicken), one vegetable (brassica), one carbohydrate (rice or potato), one fruit (banana or apple), water and vitamin supplements. If no headaches (or only one) were experienced during the last two weeks of the 3-4 week diet then the excluded foods were reintroduced sequentially at the rate of one a week and remained in the diet if no symptoms occurred. If symptoms occurred the food was withdrawn at the end of the week.

Of the 88 children who completed the diet, 78 'recovered completely' and 4 'improved greatly'. On re-introduction of one or more foods all but 8 relapsed and these 8 remained well. Forty of the improved group entered a double-blind controlled trial which provided clear evidence that a 'placebo response' was not the explanation for the symptoms. Many of the children also experienced an improvement in associated signs and symptoms including abdominal pain, diarrhoea, flatulence, behaviour disturbances, aching limbs, fits, rhinitis, recurrent mouth ulcers, vaginal discharge, asthma and eczema. In 38 patients the new diet almost completely eliminated the effects of some of the non-specific provokers of migraines such as exercise, trauma, emotional episodes, travel, bright light, heat and noise but not of perfumes and/or cigarette smoke. On re-exposure to the possible offending foods, those foods producing symptoms in the greatest number of children were cow's milk (27), egg (24), chocolate (22), orange (21), wheat (21), benzoic acid (14), cheese (13), tomato (13), tartrazine (12), rye (12), fish (9), pork (9), beef (8) and maize (8). Soya, tea, oats, goat's milk, coffee, peanuts, bacon, potato, yeast, mixed nuts, apple and peaches produced symptoms in 4-7 children. Skin prick tests and IgE antibodies were not found to be diagnostically useful in identifying causative foods.

Drs Ogle and Bullock, from Ohio State University College of Medicine, treated 322 infants under one year of age with respiratory allergy and negative inhalant skin tests by placing them on a hypoallergenic elimination diet for six weeks. The diet consisted of a meat base formula, beef, carrots, broccoli and apricots. Ninety-one per cent of the infants showed a significant improvement of respiratory symptoms which could be reproduced in 51 per cent of cases after oral food challenge. The most reactive foods were milk, egg, chocolate, soy, legumes and cereals in decreasing order.[23]

Another report from the Paediatric Clinic of the University of Parma, Italy, has also demonstrated a complete remission of skin symptoms in 12 out of 13 children with severe chronic eczema after they were placed on an elimination diet for two weeks. The major allergens in this case were also found to be milk and eggs.[24]

These studies all demonstrate how antigenic or otherwise reactive food components, notably proteins and peptides, passing through the intestinal wall of susceptible individuals and travelling through the bloodstream, may trigger immunological or non-immunological events in specific target organs such as the lungs, joints, central nervous system or skin (as well as the gut). Acute inflammatory reactions, behaviour modifications, changes in mental processes and chronic degenerative changes are just a few of the possible outcomes.

Such a concept was considered improbable in the past because it was generally assumed that all large protein molecules were broken down by digestive enzymes to yield their component amino acids before intestinal absorption. The idea is no longer far fetched and even large protein digestive enzymes (such as trysin) appear to be recirculated from the intestines to the blood stream and vice versa in both animals and humans.[25]

It is highly likely that a malfunctional intestinal screening barrier may act as a flood gate for the absorption of allergenic proteins and peptides which can subsequently give rise to one of a spectrum of different clinical disorders. In order to minimise such an adverse effect we can take the following steps:

a Remove known food offenders from a mother's diet during gestation (these are foods to which the mother is known to react in a predictable manner at any time of exposure in any quantity).

b Eat suspected foods only once every 4 days during the entire pregnancy and continue this practice throughout lactation. This minimises sensitization of the foetus in utero while still allowing limited in utero exposure.

c   Breast feed exclusively and postpone the infant's exposure to foreign proteins for at least 6 months to allow the baby's immune system and digestive system to function optimally (this takes up to 6 months).

CHAPTER 2

CONTROLLING
INTERMITTENT
FOOD INTOLERANCE
AND ADDICTION

FOOD CRAVINGS

If you eat prawns and always get hives, or oranges and predictably get a migraine, or strawberries and find yourself covered with a rash, and this always happens in a predictable fashion every time you eat the suspect food then you have a 'fixed' allergy and you are in the minority — only a small percentage of food sensitivities fall into this category. Obviously the thing to do is to completely eliminate the food from your diet.

The great majority of food intolerances are not 'fixed', they are called 'cyclic' allergies and are not consistent. One week you could react to the food and another week have no reaction at all. If you have not eaten the food for two or three weeks and suddenly consume it daily for two to three days and in large quantities you may start to react because of your increased exposure to the food. On many occasions people may only react to a food if they are *also* exposed to an inhalant allergen such as house dust, cat or dog fur, pollens or even sudden wind or temperature changes. These additional allergic factors push the person over the allergic stress threshold, ie, dairy products or house dust by themselves may give no reaction but together may cause an allergic reaction. The same applies to mental or emotional stress. Frequently an allergic manifestation will not arise until you lose your job, go through a divorce, suffer the loss of a loved one, or experience some other emotional trauma.

An overload of stress factors on the body causes it to break down under the strain – either physically, mentally or emotionally – the specific manifestation of the stress overload will vary depending on the individual.

Some of the cardinal signs of food intolerance are:

a Uncontrollable cravings for specific foods;

b Excessive quantities consumed and increased frequency of consumption of a specific food, especially during times of stress;

c A food which induces a markedly increased state of well-being like a drug-induced 'high', and which you come to depend upon.

The best test is to ask yourself which food you could not possibly do without. In nine times out of ten this food will be the culprit (or at least one of them).

A good example is the teenage boy who comes home from school irritable, aggressive and hungry and always heads for the milk in the refrigerator. After drinking a full litre the boistrous behaviour stops. American researchers have demonstrated that many juvenile delinquents consume up to six litres of milk each day. Milk craving has often been shown to result from an addictive allergy which leads to aggressive behaviour modification.[26] I have consistently found that migraine sufferers consume copious quantities of either cheese, butter, milk or other dairy products. The migraines stop only after the dairy products have been removed from the diet. Sometimes these patients can resume eating specific types of dairy products after abstaining for several months but others cannot, depending on which protein fraction is doing the damage, ie, they may be able to eat ricotta cheese which is made from the whey portion of the milk but not hard cheese, or vice versa. Some can take butter but not milk. Such specific sensitivities can only be tested after the complete withdrawal of all dairy products from their diet.

Bread is another good example of an addictive allergy. Some individuals just cannot go without bread, even for a day – toast for breakfast, sandwiches for lunch, bread with dinner. The standard reaction to the suggestion of 'no more bread' is the statement 'what is there left to eat?' This type of person can quite easily consume up to one loaf of bread a day, and it is usual to find them consuming half a loaf. If you have an abnormal craving for bread, do you also crave biscuits, cakes, pastries, cereals and wheat flour products in general, and especially at times of increased emotional stress? If you do, there is a good chance that your addictive allergy may be to 'gluten', the protein component of wheat. Gluten is also found in rye, oats and barley, however, so watch out for these foods as well.

If you crave not only bread but also vegemite, beer, wine or other yeast containing foods, there is a likelihood that you may have a yeast rather than a gluten sensitivity. Both sensitivities may occur together.

These addictive foods are always over-consumed and at frequent intervals. If you miss eating them you will start to feel bad. This is because such addictive foods act as stressors on the body in much the same way as addictive drugs such as heroine, amphetamines and nicotine. When you miss having your regular fix you start to have withdrawal symptoms just like a drug addict. Your body starts rebelling against the removal of the food on which it has come to depend.

The body fights stress, whether physical, emotional, mental or allergic by releasing specific hormones. One of these is adrenaline. The racing car driver is under acute 'stress' as he battles to take the lead at over 200km/hour, but the adrenaline burst gives him a 'high', the memory of which sends him back for more. The same may be said of the fanatical following which has arisen for computer games such as Space Invaders. Fun parlours are never empty and many children spend hours in front of their own home computers. So strong is the grip of these machines on psychological and physiological processes that children have been known to steal money from their parents just to play them. Why do some individuals sit in clubs playing the poker machines from opening time until the machines are shut off at night? The answer is addiction. The anticipation of a windfall gives a continual high mediated by hormone release within the body. This same high can be elicited by addictive foods though the effect may be more subtle. One group of hormones released when the body is placed under stress is called 'endorphins'. These are chemicals produced in the body which act on the brain in a similar fashion to opiates such as morphine. Endorphins help reduce pain perception and other symptomatic problems associated with stressors such as food allergens. They can also give some people a temporary sense of well-being and even an euphoria. This pleasant feeling has often been experienced by the long distance runner whose physiological stress (and endorphin) levels rise as the run progresses. While this process is at present little understood, it is believed that during an adverse food reaction endorphins and other opiates are released which stimulate a craving for that food. So it is not the food itself that addicts the person, it is possibly the subsequent stress-induced release of endorphin with its opiate-like effects.

As a result of this physiological response to addictive foods, the person may experience considerable swings in mood—from happy, excitable and even manic on some occasions to depressed, lethargic and tired on others. The good sense of humour today converts to an argumentative disposition tomorrow.

These mood and behaviour changes can be tracked down to the frequency of exposure to the addictive food. While the body is getting its regular 'fixes' of the specific reactant food(s) everything is fine but if it misses its fix, a good case of the blues is likely to descend and gloom takes over as the stimulating phase of addictant exposure gives way to the withdrawal phase of addictant elimination. Withold the suspect food and the body starts to rebel. This latter stage is the time when the specific food craving will be at its highest but after returning to the food, the withdrawal symptoms are replaced by the stimulating phase that is associated with exposure to the food.

A person rarely gets too far into the withdrawal phase before reaching for their reactive food. For this reason such addictive food allergies are masked. The real withdrawal symptoms are masked by eating more of the same food. During food elimination under conditions of controlled fasting, the wifhdrawal symptoms appear in full force and for the first few days you can feel quite ill. This withdrawal period called 'unmasking' can be quite traumatic and may include nausea, vomiting, diarrhoea, headaches, aching joints and muscles, fatigue, mucous discharge, breathlessness and increased heart rate, to name but a few. These symptoms may be in addition to emotional upheavals, increased sensitivity and nervousness, increased anger, irritability, argumentative nature or perhaps depression, somnolence and apathy. Watch for family arguments during this period. For some people, however, the withdrawal period may be relatively mild.

Usually after 4-5 days the symptoms subside and a marvellous sense of wellbeing, vitality and increased awareness emerges as the stressful veil of food intolerance is lifted. Note, though, at this stage re-exposure to the reactive foods will cause immediate symptoms, usually more severe than previously because the body in its new state is now exquisitely sensitive to allergens. This is the body's natural warning system starting to work properly to tell us immediately not to eat the food. Prior to the unmasking phase the body had increased its tolerance for the food and so the alarm mechanisms were shut off.

Many alternative health practitioners refer to the symptoms experienced during a fast as the 'healing crisis'. No doubt during this time not only is the body relieved of the allergic stressors but the normal digestive and other anabolic processes shut down, allowing the body to enter a rest and recuperative phase, which may also result in an internal cleansing of accumulated toxins. It is also noteworthy that hypoglycaemic (low blood sugar) patients with food intolerances feel 100 per cent better after such a fast – the hypoglycaemia is secondary to the food intolerance. Many hypoglycaemic patients have been advised not to fast as their blood sugar levels would drop even further. In the case of food intolerances, where hypoglycaemia is a secondary phenomenon, this will not occur.

As already stated the great majority of food intolerances are cyclic. They come and go depending upon the frequency and length of exposure to a particular reactive food. Seasonal fruits and vegetables can lead to an over-consumption of one or more of a family of foods for a limited period and result in a food intolerance over this period of time. For example, stone fruits such as cherries, peaches or plums may be eaten infrequently and without symptoms during the year when shipped from another country, but in the stone fruit season a sensitivity to cherries may slowly built up through constant exposure on a daily basis.

Some grain sensitive people respond well to the first 3-4 weeks of substituting whole grain brown rice for wheat on a daily basis, but after the first month rice intolerance symptoms may emerge due to the daily exposure to rice. This phenomenon is rare in the case of rice, but not so rare in the case of other gluten-containing grains such as rye, barley and oats.

Any food eaten on a daily basis may lead to intolerance depending on individual susceptibilities,and the most frequently consumed foods are the prime candidates. In Australia they are milk and wheat products—the two food types which are consumed at almost every meal, including snacks. In the US there is also a marked increase in sensitivities to corn and soya products since the rapid increase in the use of these two food stuffs in most processed foods.

Sensitivity to one food may also mean a sensitivity to other foods that belong in the same food family. A person sensitive to tomatoes may also have a sensitivity to the other members of the family, ie potatoes, eggplant, peppers (capsicum, chillies, paprika) and tobacco. But the food family concept may be over-rated as we will soon discover. In addition, there is an increased chance of an adverse food reaction the larger the amount of food consumed at a sitting. For this reason it is important to stick to moderate servings.

Unlike the 'fixed' allergies which require total elimination of the food concerned, addictive cyclic allergies can be controlled adequately after an initial unmasking elimination period simply by rotating food types so that the same foods are not eaten every day. This gives the body a break from a particular food and allows it to recuperate. It also maximises nutritional requirements when the diet is carefully balanced. Instead of eating beef every day, for example, you may eat it once a week, and on the other days rotate chicken, fish, pork, shellfish, etc. In this way the daily primary protein source comes from a different type of animal. While many people think of salad as being lettuce and tomato, the daily salad can be varied by using coleslaw one day, cucumber and grated beetroot the next, celery and watercress or bean sprouts the next, and so on.

This rotation of food types on different days will not only prevent food intolerance from developing but it also offers a more nutritionally sound diet through exposure to a greater variety of foods.

The unmasking process can also be accomplished by rotating foods without an initial specific food elimination period but the whole procedure takes longer. The advantage is that the withdrawal symptoms are far less severe and in some cases may not be evident at all.

A RE-EXAMINATION OF THE FOOD FAMILY CONCEPT

Within food families some members are more allergenic than others. In the grain family wheat is usually more allergenic than rice; in the legume family, peanuts elicit a greater number of adverse reactions than do beans; oranges cause far more problems than grapefruit or lemons and are a well-known precipitant of migraines; eggs are notorious allergens for infants and younger children but chicken is not, and in some cases the egg yolk is well tolerated but not the white. It is common to find cow's milk a major problem but not necessarily beef or veal and so on.

The observations indicate that single foods may cause problems *which are not shared by other members of the same family of foods*. This is one of the most important points to consider when discussing cyclic allergies where daily exposure to a specific food, such as peanuts, is more detrimental than daily exposure to a wide variety of foods within the same family. For example, alfalfa sprouts, lima beans, carob, chickpeas, lentils, gardenpeas and soybean products or soy milk eaten one at a time on consecutive days will not elicit the same adverse reaction as eating peanuts every day. All of these foods are in the legume family, but each type of food is rotated so that a single food is not consumed on a daily basis. Sensitivities may extend to all members of the family but this depends upon whether the allergenic components are present in all members of that family or in all food products derived from that family. If a person has a gluten sensitivity he/she must not only abstain from wheat and wheat products but also barley, oats and rye which are also gluten-containing foods. However, some individuals who cannot tolerate wheat find no problem with barley or oats. Adverse reactions to members of the grain family are not necessarily due to the gluten proteins. For this reason there are rare individuals who cannot tolerate rice but can eat wheat.

MAJOR PLANT FOOD FAMILIES (common items)

Grass Family
barley, corn, millet, oats, rice, rye, sugar cane, molasses, wheat.

Legume Family
alfalfa, carob, chickpea (garbanzo), lentil, pea, peanut, lima beans, mung beans, kidney beans, soybean, lecithin.

Mustard Family
broccoli, Brussels sprouts, cabbage, cauliflower, horseradish, mustard greens, mustard seed, radish, swede (rutabaga), turnip, watercress.

Carrot Family
carrot, celery, parsley, parsnip.

Cashew Family
cashew, mango, pistachio.

Potato Family (Nightshade)
eggplant (aubergine), capsicum (red or green pepper), cayenne, chili, paprika, potato, tobacco, tomato.

Gourd Family
cucumber, gherkin, rockmelon (cantaloupe), honeydew melon, pumpkin, squash (marrow), zucchini (courgettes), watermelon.

Lily Family
asparagus, chives, garlic, leek, onion, shallot.

Palm Family
coconut, cofa, date, sago.

Citrus Family
grapefruit, lemon, lime, orange, tangerine, kumquat.

Rose Family
apple, pear, quince, almond, apricot, cherry, peach, plum, berries.

Buckwheat Family
buckwheat,
rhubarb.

Grape Family
grape, currant, raisin, wine.

Composite Family
artichoke, camomile, chicory, dandelion, endive, lettuce, safflower oil, sunflower oil.

Custard Apple Family
custard apple, paw paw (papaya).

Goosefoot
beets, chard, spinach.

Ginger Family
cardamon, ginger, turmeric.

Dr N. Childers[27] has maintained that arthritis is basically due to hypersensitive reactions to the nightshade family. Thousands of patients recovered when they removed tomato, potato, peppers, eggplants, and tobacco from their diet. However, to interpret Childers results as meaning that no other foods are involved is to make the same mistake that Feingold made in thinking that hyperkinetic behaviour was mainly due to salicylates and chemical additives in foods. We now know that many other dietary and environmental factors are involved. Marshall Mandell,[28] like Childers, found a large body of rheumatic sufferers allergic to nightshades (50% reacted to potato and 30% to tomato using systematic sublingual provocation tests) but he also found in the same group of patients a staggering 73% reaction to soybean, 36% to peanuts, 60% allergic to egg or milk, 50% to yeast or beef and over 40% to chicken or mould. These results suggest that soybeans have a greater allergenic potential for arthritic patients in the US than the nightshade family, possibly due to the rapid increase in the use of soya products in American processed foods over recent years. This is another example of increased exposure to specific foods relating to food sensitivity. Of even greater importance was the finding that patients reacting to one member of a family of foods did not necessarily react to other members of the same family.

Mandell and Conte[28] examined the reactions of 30 volunteer arthritic subjects to a series of double-blind sublingual challenges with unidentified test solutions containing the major allergens: mould, apple, auto exhaust, beef, chicken, chocolate, coffee, corn, egg, ethanol, house dust, lettuce, milk, natural gas, orange, pork, potato, peanut, soy, sugar, tea, tobacco, tomato, wheat, and bakers yeast. After 2,610 double-blind provocation tests they found an 'absence of a common family-wide allergen that would be characterised by allergic cross-reactivity between members of the same taxonomic group . . .' Fourteen patients reacting to soybeans did not react to peanuts which are in the same family. Of the cereal grains, corn, sugar and wheat, three subjects only reacted to corn, four only reacted to cane sugar and five reacted to wheat but had no reaction to either corn or sugar. Eight milk sensitive patients had no reaction to beef, while six beef sensitive subjects did not react to milk. Both of these foods are bovine in origin. Of 10 individuals who did react to both milk and beef, the same symptoms were not elicited by each food possibly because the beef muscle and milk proteins are different and thus have different allergenic qualities. The same findings were evident for the chicken/egg allergens where five chicken allergic patients failed to react to egg and 10 egg sensitive patients showed no reaction to chicken. In the fungus family five mould sensitive subjects failed to react to yeast and six with a yeast allergy had no reaction to mould and only five out of 15 potato reactors were allergic to tomatoes.

These results confirm my own findings and further provide evidence for the lack of a universal food family allergen in all food families tested. Adverse reactions frequently arise from a specific food but not necessarily from other food members of the same family. When adverse reactions to members of the same family were observed, each food gave rise to different symptoms, indicating that different allergens were involved.

The same line of reasoning explains why some wheat sensitive patients can eat oats and barley. It simply means that their sensitivity is *not* to, say, alpha-gliaden (a gluten protein), it is to some other reactive protein present in wheat but not in oats or barley. Alternatively the chemical sprays, or additives involved in the processing of wheat may be different from those used for processing oats or barley.

It is of course, still possible to have a patient react to soybeans and peanuts which are in the same family but it is more likely in many instances that adverse reactions arise not from a common food family allergen, but from distinctly different reactant molecules which just happen to exist in many foods of the same family but are not necessarily uniquely family related.

These results confirm many of the seemingly inconsistent observations I have found in my own patients who could not, for example, tolerate eggs but could eat chicken (ie the same animal) with no ill effects. I rarely found beef intolerance in milk sensitive individuals. This apparent contradiction, namely that different edible parts of the same animal do not induce the same allergenic reaction, is due to differences in allergenicity between the proteins found in, say, the milk (such as casein, lactoglobulin etc) and those found in edible tissues from the animal (such as the major connective tissue protein collagen). This point is not always emphasised in books which discuss the allergic properties of whole families of foods. In fact, throughout my diet plans I have included different members of the same family more frequently than advocated in standard four day rotation diets which state that any one item from a single food family should not be consumed more than once within a four day period. Carrots, parsley and turnips are all in the same family but can usually be eaten every other day (ie. carrots day 1, parsley day 3, turnips day 5). This, of course, represents only a two-day rotation. Some individuals can even eat them on a daily basis. It should be pointed out at this stage that it is easier to eat vegetable families more frequently than it is to eat meets or grains. According to clinical observations lamb in Australia causes far fewer adverse reactions than beef and can be tolerated far more frequently than beef products. Pumpkin can be tolerated much more readily than potatoes. Many rotation diets are far too restrictive because they do not take these observations into account and stick rigidly to the food family concept.

Cow's milk intolerance is fairly widespread in our society but this does not automatically mean that a milk intolerant person cannot eat dairy products. Milk, yoghurt and products which include cow's milk such as icecream, custards, junkets, pudding, etc all contain lactose (which is the natural milk sugar) and are not tolerated by those with lactose intolerance in any large amounts. But even lactose intolerant individuals may be able to take small quantities of lactose containing products as there is a threshold for lactose intolerance. As long as the lactose level in the diet is below this threshold, there is no adverse reaction. This contrasts sharply with a milk allergy due to one or more of the milk proteins which may give severe reactions after consuming only a small amount. A lactose intolerant person may be able to handle hard cheese which contains only trace amounts of lactose. Frequently cream cheeses can also be tolerated as they vary in lactose content, but should be checked with the manufacturer before use. For some unknown reason certain lactose intolerant people can tolerate yoghurt, which does contain lactose. The main point to remember with lactose intolerance is to eat small portions only of suspected foods.

The most common problem with cow's milk intolerance is an allergic reaction to one (or more) of the five milk proteins. The most frequent offender is a protein called beta-lactoglobulin. This protein is not present in human milk. Other studies have indicated that a major milk protein, casein, may also cause an adverse food reaction. If casein is the suspect, ricotta cheese may be tolerated. Ricotta cheese is made by separating the curds (containing the casein) from the whey (which contains soluble proteins including beta-lactoglobulin). When the whey is acidified these soluble proteins such as the albumins precipitate to form the bulk of the ricotta cheese. If lactalbumin is the problem you may tolerate the casein in hard cheeses. It is still, however, wise to check with the manufacturing process if you are not making the cheese yourself. If you suspect dairy products, separate them into groups and test them individually in the following order: hard cheeses, ricotta, cream, butter, milk, yoghurt.

Sometimes the allergenic qualities of milk can be removed by extended boiling. In this way the heat applied is sufficient to change the shape of the allergenic protein molecules ('denatures' the protein) which makes them inactive. Heat-treated whey has the least allergenic properties.

Another way to reduce the possible allergic reaction associated with grains, seeds or legumes is to sprout them. Not only are sprouts more easily digested, but the protein composition of the seed changes during the sprouting process and this may remove potential allergenic proteins. In the legume family, for example, alfalfa seeds and lentils are an obvious choice for sprouting, but make sure they have not been sprayed with any chemicals.

CHAPTER 3

SUGAR AND
FOOD
INTOLERANCE

SUGAR AND COMPLEX CARBOHYDRATES

Two of the most common questions asked about diets are a) whether sugar is permitted, and b) what is the relationship between hypoglycaemia (low blood sugar) and food intolerance.

Despite the popular view that sugars are a necessary component of our diet we can get all the sugars we need from starches contained in the complex carbohydrates of legumes, vegetables and grains. Many people are not aware of the fact that all starches found in foods are converted to sugars in our body. In many respects, this is the best way of obtaining such sugars because they are released slowly from the starch and give rise to a more gradual increase in blood sugar level. This 'slow release' phenomenon is helped further by eating whole unprocessed complex carbohydrates which are high in fibre.[29] Obviously the most popular way of obtaining sugar is from the sugar bowl, confectionaries, cakes, biscuits, icecream, soft drinks and so on. Another way people increase their sugar levels without realizing it is by consuming copious quantities of pure fruit juices. Fruit juice may be 100% natural but it is still loaded with sugar and can cause rapid elevations and subsequent compensatory falls in blood sugar. You would never eat 10-20 apples a day – but may drink the equivalent amount of juice. This is not good for your health. Eat the fruit and you'll eat the right quantity – your stomach will tell you. When you drink pure juices always dilute them 1 part to at least two parts water or mineral water. Very important neuronal pathways are triggered off by the natural pressure from the chewing action of the jaw (the temperomandibular joint). This pathway is activated appropriately if we eat unrefined whole foods – but not if we drink the juices of the foods or alternatively eat heavily refined foods. Note how much longer it takes to eat whole grain foods compared with refined flour products like cakes and biscuits. Note the difference in time to eat a plate of white rice compared with brown rice. This increase in time is vital – it means you chew more, secrete greater quantities of salivary and digestive enzymes and have enhanced digestive capacity. More importantly, you eat less because you feel fuller more quickly. On the inside there is another advantage already mentioned. The starch from whole grains, legumes and vegetables is converted to sugar and released into the blood stream much more slowly than equivalent amounts of refined carbohydrates or sugar and leads to a stable and sustained rise in blood sugar.[30] The cellular structure of whole foods acts as a slow release capsule. This is also what happens when we eat whole fruit compared with drinking the juice of the fruit.[31] The whole fruit gives a much slower rise in blood sugar and hence stimulates less of an insulin response. So the nature and form of the food we eat (ie whole versus processed) can affect our blood sugar levels and hormone regulation.[32,33] In the state of optimal health, blood glucose and other indices fluctuate minimally and we should aim to keep the balance that way by the appropriate choice of food which has undergone minimal processing.

As well as sugar substitutes such as cyclamate and saccharine, there are several natural sugar alternatives to sucrose, the common table sugar. Unfortunately, these all have serious drawbacks. Sucrose alone has a long list of negative factors associated with its consumption which includes increased insulin and corticosteroid levels, increased 'stickiness' of blood platelets, and reductions in the level of high density lipoprotein cholesterol (which protects against heart disease), glucose intolerance, retinopathy and nephropathy.[35] Fructose is not much better as it has been shown to increase uric acid, lactic acid, cholesterol and triglyceride levels in the blood stream.[36, 37] Sucrose is actually 50 per cent fructose. Lactose (milk sugar) can stir up lactose intolerance which appears to be present in over 54 per cent of the world's population and perhaps 30 million in the US.[34] Sorbitol can cause diarrhoea in children[38] and problems with eyesight (animal studies). Ultimately glucose has fewer problems than any of the other sugars and is the only food for the brain and nerves but of course, if taken in large amounts can elicit a large insulin response which can cause reactive hypolgycaemia (ie low blood sugar). So it is far better to get your sugar from vegetables and fruit. If you are going to use a sweetener, within the framework of your permitted foods use honey, carob or glucose. Honey and carob contain fructose but they also contain other trace nutrients involved in the metabolic pathways of fructose metabolism and are most likely less harmful in this respect than refined sucrose or fructose. Many of the bad effects of sugar may well result from the removal of the trace nutrients which were originally present in the initial unprocessed state. The B vitamins, thiamin and niacin and trace elements, chromium, zinc and manganese in particular help to optimally metabolise sugar in the body.

HYPOGLYCAEMIA AND FOOD INTOLERANCE

Hypoglycaemia simply means low blood sugar and apart from various organic causes such as Addison's disease, hypopituitarism and insulinoma is thought to be more frequently caused by the massive intake of sugar and foods containing sugar or refined carbohydrates. As the blood sugar quickly rises a substance called insulin is released from the pancreas and immediately undertakes the task of removing sugar from the blood stream and shunting it into the cells of the body. This can reduce the level of sugar in the blood if too much insulin is released. This is most likely to happen if massive amounts of sugar are rapidly absorbed in any form. So eating large quantities of sugar can actually lower blood sugar levels causing hypoglycaemia. Another common cause of hypoglycaemia is any chronic stress on the body that tends to over-tax the adrenal glands which secrete adrenaline and cortisone (the stress hormones) into the blood stream. Initially, adrenaline and cortisone tend to increase the blood sugar level, which produces extra energy for the body to cope with the stressful condition. The sugar level can quickly drop however if the adrenal glands start to become exhausted due to chronic stress. The body just cannot cope adequately with the stressful situation. This is especially the case with food allergies or intolerances where the reactive food acts as a stressor on the body in much the same way as a fright, an accident, a death in the family, financial difficulties, marital problems and the like.

In fact if blood sugar levels are measured directly after a person has eaten a food to which they are sensitive, there is frequently a drop in blood sugar or sometimes a rapid rise.[39] These sudden changes in blood sugar levels have nothing to do with whether a person has eaten sugar or not. They are physiological changes which reflect stress on the body and will readily occur after the person has eaten allergenic foods such as beef, egg, wheat, cheese or other protein allergens or reactive fragments which cause the body to swing into its specific metabolic state of red alert for handling stress.

This low blood sugar condition will not respond to the elimination of sugar and junk food, though the person will certainly feel better without them. What is needed in this case is for the offending food or foods to be traced and eliminated. These unsuspected foods cause continuing lethargy, weakness, fatigue and tiredness. Even though the person may be taking in a lot of sugar, coffee, alcohol, etc, this may be solely to get a burst of energy to compensate for the real cause of the problem. In this way an excessive sugar craving may be a secondary phenomenon to the real culprit – a food intolerance.

Many of my patients had previously given up sugar and other stimulants after reading about the problem of hypoglycaemia and also changed to a more healthy diet to find that they felt only marginally better. The basic problem persisted. After specific food elimination and subsequent rechallenge with the same food at a later date they were found to have one or more food sensitivities which were causing all their hypoglycaemic symptoms and which invariably disappeared after the appropriate dietary manipulation.

ALL STRESSORS EXACERBATE FOOD INTOLERANCE

It is most important to see all forms of stress as playing a role in stimulating or exacerbating food sensitivities. All forms of stress place an extra load on the adrenal glands, the insulin secreting glands of the pancreas, the digestive system, the immune system and the nervous system. These systems work together with other biological support systems to protect us from viruses, bacteria, inhalant allergens, food allergens and other foreign invaders of the body. Stress can lead to malfunction of one or all of these systems.

I have seen a patient suddenly come down with rheumatoid arthritis after a car accident, another with eczema after a marriage separation and several with asthma after emotional upheavals at home. Frequently such patients start to complain of one or more food intolerances at the same time. Others with relatively minor food sensitivities have suddenly found that they have contracted severe multiple food sensitivities immediately following an emotional crisis point in their life. This may manifest as eczema, psosriasis, arthritis, asthma, migraine, gastrointestinal disturbances or even mental health disorders. In fact, the potential for such disorders was possibly always present but held in check by the natural protective mechanisms of the body such as the immune system, adrenal glands, etc until the stress overload became too great and suddenly a minor subclinical condition becomes a fully blown clinical situation as the multiple stress forces finally overwhelm the body's natural buffers.

In other words food intolerance manifestations are frequently an accumulative effect of many stress components which can include not only food but also emotional and mental stressors; family disharmony, financial difficulties, poor exercise and eating habits, lack of sleep, sudden changes in weather conditions (humidity, temperature, rain, fog), chemical sensitivity, physical trauma, exhaustion, car accidents, crash diets, malnutrition and a whole range of seemingly unrelated factors. The cumulative effect of several of these stress factors can suddenly precipitate a food sensitivity even though the food has been eaten for years with no obvious untoward effects. What happens in this situation is that the total stress load reaches its breaking point and something has to give. The extra stress factor is the straw that breaks the camel's back. One or more of the many distinct physiological buffer systems of the body can no longer cope adequately. At this stage the allergenic potential of a food acting on a genetic susceptibility or an in utero derived weakness, may suddenly manifest due to the stress induced changes in the body's protective biological mechanism.

This allergenic potential does not have to express. Food intolerance is not a fait accompli. The condition has been compared to that of a loaded gun where the bullets are the allergens and the pulled trigger the external stressors, such as emotional trauma. The gun can do no harm so long as the trigger is not pulled and the gun is well looked after. By analogy the allergic gun is fired when the pressure on the trigger becomes too great due to the burden of accumulated stress factors.

This is why we so frequently hear of how wonder cures have occured through stress management programs, relaxation therapy, specific diets and nutrition supplementation, meditation, mind control techniques, yoga and various sporting activities such as swimming, jogging and other aerobic exercises, all of which reduce the total stress load on a person and also illustrate that there are many different approaches toward the treatment of the same problem.

Aerobic exercise, for example, reduces acidosis, pumps fresh oxygenated blood to all tissues, exercises muscles, normalises bowel movements, moves lymphatic fluid and revs up sluggish metabolic machinery. Meditation and other relaxation techniques slow down the thought process and increase awareness, hence take much of the emotional and mental energy drain off the body, ie feelings of anger, hate, jealousy, and greed. Worry and anxiety are considerably reduced by being cut off at the source. These positive activities all tend to reduce the stress hormone levels and slow down the nervous system in general. A person can then respond to the environment in a more centred and controlled manner when free of exaggerated emotions and useless internal dialogue. This means more efficient spontaneous activities, greater clarity of thought and an associated gearing down of the metabolic machinery that has been running overtime under stress conditions.

So the correct way to tackle these problems is firstly by trying to remove the obvious sources of the stress. Here, counselling may be of prime importance and relaxation therapy, meditation, yoga, aerobic exercises, a good long rest with plenty of sleep or perhaps a holiday, may all be factors to consider. At the same time the apparent food sensitivities can be reduced by adhering to the specific diet plans outlined in this book. Vitamin, mineral and enzyme therapy may be necessary to boost immune function, digestion and general energy levels, but above all there should be no stress imposed by this type of program itself.

CHAPTER 4

CRITICAL
STRESS
COMPONENTS

THE STRESS OF THE ANTI-ALLERGY PROGRAMS

Frequently, the anxious patient suffering from food intolerances is made decidedly worse by the stress induced from adhering strictly to an eliminating diet in which only a few foods are permitted. The patient worries that he or she is eating the wrong foods or that X-brand of soy milk had lactose in it or that Mrs Smith will not possibly understand the reasons for her refusing the food when she attends the dinner party next Friday. After a while the new diet and the associated changes in lifestyle start to become some strange new religious dogma with fanaticism, guilt, fear and anxiety emerging.

This must not happen on any account. Work out the specific life style changes and diet – then forget it. Don't dwell on it, don't talk about it, just do it to the best of your ability. If one day you find yourself compulsively eating an ice cream or chocolate biscuit and nothing is going to stop you – then enjoy it! You'll do yourself more harm by punishing yourself with feelings of guilt while you eat it and then by continuing to feel guilty for weeks after.

If you must have ideas about the diet and your new found activities, think positively. Visualise yourself in the future as being full of energy and vitality, perhaps having lost those few extra kilos. See the diet as a fun experiment with foods. Try to look on it as a new and creative activity involving the changing of your lifestyle for the better. If you do not always achieve what you set out to accomplish think then only of the ground that you have already made and of your achievements.

It is always advisable to remove your allergenic foods from the household, but if this is impossible because of family pressures there is one good way of side-tracking yourself when the urge to indulge in a huge sandwich of thick peanut butter, honey and chocolate gets hold of you. Replace the negative urge with a positive one. For example, as your body pulls you towards the refrigerator wherein lurks the forbidden food, immediately turn off your thoughts, and according to a precalculated action, head for your jogging gear, move your body out of the door and before you've started to think again, you're happily jogging down the street with the good feeling inside that you have converted a potentially damaging activity into a highly productive positive one. Try this concept of converting negative activities into positive ones in other areas related to your new program.

It is also of great benefit to have the entire family or household members embark on the program together, if not the entire program, at least the diet. In this way food preparation becomes much simpler as everyone is eating the same foods and you also get a little more sympathy and support if all members of the entire group are 'in it together'. Trying to prepare three different meals at once can be one of the major stress factors mentioned.

THE LOST ART OF EATING

Many aspects of food intolerance have nothing whatsoever to do with the actual food and are more related to attitude and lifestyle.

We have already discussed the importance of food 'form' and recognized the value of eating the whole grain rather than its flour products or eating the piece of fruit instead of drinking its juice. Of equal importance is the manner in which we eat the food. Mealtime should be one of the stress-free times of the day. All aspects related to eating a meal can have a very powerful though secondary effect on a food intolerance.

One of the greatest contributors to poor digestion, gastrointestinal disorders, obesity and a wide range of clinical conditions is overeating. We all eat too much. This fact alone places enormous strain on digestive enzymes in the stomach, pancreas and small intestines. Just by cutting down on our food intake we can double the effectiveness of our entire digestive system. We would never dream of doubling the maximum load of a washing machine especially if the washing powder was already limited and the machine suffering from the wear and tear of many years of faithful service. The outcome would most certainly be a washing basket full of wet half-cleaned fabrics which would have to go back into the machine.

Unfortunately, our food doesn't get a second chance after being swallowed. We just get incomplete digestion and the dumping of semi-digested food proteins (as well as carbohydrates and fats) into the small intestines where protein breakdown products are absorbed. These half-digested protein fragments, called peptides, as well as whole undigested proteins may be the allergens for many people with food intolerances. If possible also try to avoid excessively hot or cold food and beverages. These cause shocks to the digestive system.

One popular activity at the dinner table is 'food bolting', a competitive situation where participants proceed to devour the entire contents of the plate in the shortest possible time and with the least number of chews per mouthful.

Nearly one third of carbohydrate digestion can occur in the mouth by salivary enzymes if we give it a chance. By not chewing well we place an additional load on the enzymes of the pancreas and small intestines which then have to handle what the mouth failed to cope with. Incidentally, missing teeth, malocclusion and temporomand-ibular joint problems will exacerbate an existing food sensitivity, so it is always wise to check with a dentist if you feel you may have such a problem.

When we eat it is best if we refrain from watching television, reading a newspaper or book, or listening to a conversation on the radio. The stress of noise can hinder digestion. For this reason it is advisable to talk quietly and only if necessary. Don't feel threatened by silence at the table. This is how it should be. Refrain from arguing and never teach children table manners during the meal. Wait until after or explain table etiquette before the meal. Don't jump up in the middle of a meal. Take the phone off the hook. Give yourself plenty of time to eat. If you only have five minutes before leaving in a rush you are better to wait until a relaxed interval presents itself later in the day. This is especially important in the morning. If you never have time for breakfast get up a little earlier and make time. A relaxed breakfast will more than compensate for the lost sleep. It is more important that we don't eat while walking, driving or performing some physical activity. The only situation more harmful to our digestion is eating while we are emotionally disturbed, as may occur in the middle of a heated family argument or when waiting for a special phone call. When we are upset our digestion switches off.

When we sit down at the table sit up straight with both feet on the floor with spine away from the back of the chair. Correct posture is most important for good digestion. Eat gracefully with small mouthfuls and put your fork on the plate between mouthfuls rather than loading up immediately for the next one. Wait until the last mouthful is swallowed before starting to prepare for the next. Instead of thinking about this and that, put all of your attention on the eating process. When you eat just eat. Don't prepare tomorrow's work timetable. Taste the food flavours, the texture of each mouthful, smell the odours, feel the food in your mouth, your teeth chewing, tongue and lips moving. Stop thinking and start to eat with more awareness.

While all of these points may seem obvious, rather simplistic and even somewhat old-fashioned to some, their importance cannot be overstated.

THE STRESS OF USELESS THOUGHTS

During this entire program remember you are changing your lifestyle as well as your diet. This should include the search for balance, harmony and equanimity. Do not overdo your exercise, eat moderate amounts of food, don't be an extremist. Try to aim for a good balance of mental and physical activity. If you sit in an office all day using your mind for work matters you must balance this mental excess sometime during the day with increased physical activity, especially aerobic exercises. When we think, plan, calculate, worry or indulge in any other extensive mental activity we tend to take shallow breaths and depending on the nature and extent of the mental activity we may even hold our breath without realizing it. This is why the person who is obviously under stress will suddenly take a deep breath or sigh at various intervals. They have been suffering from oxygen starvation. So exercises the body aerobically if your lifestyle requires large bursts of mental activity or when much of the day is spent daydreaming. Idle thoughts of the past or future can really zap our energy. Have you ever wondered why you can spend a whole day doing practically nothing and reach the end feeling exhausted? This is largely due to the energy draining nature of our incessant thoughts during the day—all our secret desires, dislikes, failures, successes, arguments from the past, rehashes of verbal interactions with people, planning the evening dinner, wondering what movie to see, deciding whether to return the broken toaster still under warranty, working out how to cancel Thursday's dental appointment without offending the dentist and so on. These are the types of mental stressors which account for an unaccountably tiring day.

In addition to physical exercise, as a balancing activity, it is also most beneficial to try to catch yourself in the act of daydreaming. When you do, consciously stop this energy draining and useless activity, and immediately shift your attention to your surroundings. Start observing any close object or something in your immediate environment. Let your vision seek out some distant point and hold it in your gaze. Start listening with close attention to any sounds. See how many different sounds you can hear, especially those coming from far way. Feel your body, clothes, shoes, breathing, the wind, etc. Smell your environment, those many odours or fragrances. Actually taste your food and distinguish different flavours.

All these activities of the senses we usually perform without awareness. We can actually eat an entire meal without knowing what we have eaten, we can go for a walk in a beautiful place without seeing anything, we can have a shower without really feeling the water and its heat, the soap on our body or the slippery quality of the tiles we stand on. We can drive the car and react to traffic conditions with no real awareness or sense that we are actually there driving the car. We act most of the time like machines on automatic. Only in times of crisis does everything come into clear focus. During most other times we are not really here. We are off in our private thoughts, slowly draining ourselves of energy as the central nervous system devours our body stores of glucose. We can actually consume a major portion of our body sugar supplies in this way – not by walking, running or working, but by useless mental activity. So try to use the senses more – start seeing, hearing, smelling, tasting and feeling. *You can't think and consciously use your senses at the same instant.* You can't think and see a flower. If you have thoughts about the flower, you have not actually seen its redness, or its texture. If you are thinking how nice it would look in a bowl you have stopped seeing it. It is also important when using your senses not to judge or compare the things you're seeing or listening to. Don't have any concepts about them. Just observe and listen, no thoughts, no concepts, no mental images. This art of observation is a stress-free state. Try it and watch the difference in the quality of your day. You will get to the end of it with infinitely more energy. Of course this advice should also be applied while carrying out your aerobic exercises. Feel your body jumping, listen to the sound of your breath exhaling, watch other people or objects around you. Don't plan the evening dinner, or worry about the parking meter running out of money or whether the colour of your gym suit should have been blue instead of red. If you can give all your attention to what is at hand, if you can act in the present moment entirely you can eliminate a large proportion of the major stress factors in your life.

Try to talk less, try to listen more. When someone is speaking to you, how many times do you only hear the first five words before your thoughts take over?

These concepts are vitally important. Practice the ideas outlined above. The real source of so much of our stress arises from our inner world – you cannot just blame your foods. You can change the entire way your body reacts to foods by controlling the source of inner stressors.

CHEMICAL SUSCEPTIBILITY

Hidden chemical sensitivities frequently add to or exacerbate food intolerances.[40,41] Exposure to chemicals in one form or another in our society is almost unavoidable, but we should at least be aware of the major sources in our home and at our place of employment.

During the first month of the diet plan keep such exposures to an absolute minimum.

Artificial flavours, colourings and preservatives have been omitted from all the diet plans but exposure to insecticides and other sprays associated with fruit and vegetables are quite likely. Inquire whether animal foods have been treated with hormones or antibiotics and try to secure naturally raised produce. Buy deep sea fish, which are not polluted rather than estuary fish. Thorough washing or rubbing of fruit with a dry tea towel will help to remove waxes and sprays or you may decide to buy organic foods, which are more expensive but are free from sprays. Discontinue buying aerosol products, highly perfumed petroleum based cosmetics, printed toilet paper and paper towels. Suspect products which directly contact your skin such as bleaches, dyes, disinfectants, detergents, anti-perspirant deodorants, hair sprays, perfumes, lip sticks, mascara, face creams, after shave lotions, nail polish, mouthwashes, perfumed soaps, shampoos, toothpaste, medications, mineral oil, body creams and lotions. Use natural soaps and cosmetics made with more natural ingredients. Avoid buying synthetic clothes made of polyesters. You are better to choose natural fibres. Be careful of waterproofing, permanent pressing, dry cleaning and mothproofing with camphor balls. Plastics can be another source of contamination. Watch out for clear food wrapping material and black plastic-like handles on pots and pans which are made from formaldehyde and phenol. These tend to let out toxins when heated. Replace aluminium cookware with stainless steel and avoid teflon coating.

Other major sources of chemical contamination in the home include shoe polish, floor polishes and cleaners, furniture polish, car polish, gas stoves and heaters, kerosene, varnish, carpet shampoos, rubber backing on carpets, paint fumes, oven cleaners, newsprint and felt-tip pens. Some people are also adversely effected by the positive ions generated from televisions, fluorescent lights and air conditioners. Water deionisers can purify chlorinated water.

At all times keep your house as clean as possible to minimise house dust. Keep it well ventilated, shake the mats and rugs regularly and sun sheets and blankets. Attend to any damp areas which may harbour mold. If you need to refurnish or redecorate your home use natural fibres for carpets, curtains, and upholstery. Paints and construction materials should also be chosen carefully.

Your place of employment may also be an important source of chemical exposure. Some occupations have greater risks associated with them than others. These include potters, printers, artists, garage attendants, chemists, plasterers, painters and all those working in direct contact with chemicals. Exposures may come from solvents, gases, petrochemical products and even photocopy machines. Air pollution is a major problem for some people especially car exhaust fumes which may induce nausea or headaches in some susceptible individuals before they even get to work. A vacation from home and/or work can often remove you from the chemical source for a brief period and alert you to its identity on your return. With a little thought, careful planning and perhaps reorganising, many of the previously unsuspected sources of chemical contamination can be identified and either replaced by more natural materials or eliminated completely from both the home and the work place.

The research into hyperactivity in children has come along way since Ben Feingold's work on salicylates and food additives. According to Dr Joseph McGovern[42] who specializes in the field of allergy and clinical ecology, three quarters of hyperactive children have been found to be sensitive to petrocarbons. The major chemcials involved appear to be aerosols, diesel fumes, formaldehyde, hydrocarbons, paint fumes, and petrol. When one group of 13 hyperkinetic children were exposed to various chemical solutions each child sustained an average of seven hyperkinetic reactions. The following is the percentage frequency of positive responses in the children: acetylsalicylate (aspirin) 80%, ethanol 70%, dopamine, noradrenaline, histamine 50%, indole 36%, ascorbic acid 33%, sugar and phenylalanine 30%, uric acid, corn, beef, eggs 25%, cat hair and house dust 10%.

Such results demonstrate that many drugs and phenolic food substances may produce hyperactivity in children as well as food allergens. Fifty-seven per cent of these children reacted to challenges with phenolic neurotransmitters such as dopamine and noradrenaline and all children displayed immunological abnormalities in the blood (ie, elevated histamine and prostaglandins, depressed serotonin and abnormal complement and immune complex formation.[43]

TESTS FOR FOOD INTOLERANCE

Having examined many of the contributing factors to food intolerance, let's now have a look at some commonly available tests that you can have carried out through your doctor, and also some that you can do at home.

The two most common pathology tests are the cytotoxic food allergy test and the radio allergosorbent test (RAST) both of which have limitations. There are other tests such as the skin (scratch) test and intradermal testing, but these are not as appropriate for the testing of foods and will not be discussed here. Provocative sublingual testing, serial dilation and neutralisation techniques can be discussed with your doctor.

CHAPTER 5

TESTS
FOR FOOD
INTOLERANCE

THE CYTOTOXIC FOOD ALLERGY TEST

This is a test where the patient's blood is exposed to potential allergenic foods. A sample of blood is taken and the white blood cells (called polymorphonuclear leukocytes) are separated from the red cells using a centrifuge. A suspension of these cells is then placed on a microscope slide which has a thin coating of a specific food extract on the surface. Over 100 different foods (or chemicals) may be tested in this way. Cellular changes in the white blood cells on exposure to these allergens are viewed under the microscope and graded slight, moderate or severe. Sometimes the blood cells actually swell up and break open during a severe reaction. Four days before the test, patients should discontinue the use of steroid medications such as cortisone (under the supervision of their doctor), and make sure no antihistamines, decongestants, vitamin or herbal preparations are taken within 48 hours of the test. Food and beverages should also be discontinued 12 hours before the test, with the exception of distilled, spring or mineral water.

This test has several disadvantages and I find its main use is to uncover a possible food sensitivity that has been missed after dietary manipulation and food challenge.

The controversy surrounding this test stems from the inconsistency of the test results obtained. False positive (and negative) test results may occur. If the reactive food has not been consumed within several weeks before testing, false negative results may occur. So patients should eat a wide variety of all potential allergens before the test.

Of course, this is still no guarantee that all the problem foods have actually been included. If you have been on a dairy-free diet for six months the chances of picking up a milk allergy may be slim. You are also most likely to miss seasonal food allergens which appear in the diet for a limited time only each year. The frequency of reactive food consumption before the test may also alter the test results. Consuming a food once per week may give a different result from twice per day. The other disadvantage is that the test foods may not be the same molecules that actually pass into the body to cause an adverse reaction. After a potentially reactive food protein has undergone digestion it may no longer be allergenic for the patient. Hence testing of the initial food may give a false positive reaction. The cooking and digestive processes may also remove the allergenic propensity of a food. On the other hand it is equally possible that a non-reactive food may become allergenic after the digestive enzymes have worked on it. Such reactive peptides have been demonstrated in enzymatic digests of beef, milk and wheat. The other criticism of the test is that symptoms cannot be reproduced by the test. In other words, despite the reactions of the white cells with various food extracts, there is still no relationship between the foods and patient symptoms (as is the case with provocative food testing).

The test may still be useful for the reason previously given but the limitations must be kept in mind. The other advantages of the test are the minimal time required and the lack of discomfort for the patient. This is especially important when testing psychiatric patients. It is also safe and objective from the patient's point of view, though these test results are totally dependent on the accuracy of the laboratory technician and in this respect they are subjective. There is no standardisation between laboratories.

RAST (RADIO ALLERGOSORBENT TEST)

Another commonly used test for food allergies is RAST. Using the patient's blood sample this test measures the reaction of IgE antibodies with specific food antigens (ie allergenic food fragments, usually peptides or proteins). Any positive result obtained using this test is completely reliable. If a positive reaction is found to wheat then the patient is sure that IgE antibodies are present though this may not necessarily coincide with clinical symptoms.

Only IgE mediated reactions are measured, not reactions with other immunoglobulins IgA, M,D and G which may also be involved in adverse food reactions. For this reason the test may give false negative results. The patient may have a food allergy which is mediated by one of the other immunoglobulins or may even have a food intolerance which is not mediated by immunological mechanisms at all, such as those involving prostaglandins – such reactions will not show up with the RAST.

In 1978 Ronald Trites found that two-thirds of a group of hyperactive children had elevated IgE antibodies to one or more of 42 foods tested by RAST. When the RAST positive foods were withdrawn from the children's diet over a three-week period there was a 20 per cent improvement in hyperactivity rating. A more predictable reduction in migraines was discovered by Dr Jean Monro[22] when RAST positive foods were withdrawn from patients' diets. Beneficial results were demonstrated in over two-thirds of the patients studied.

Other tests which have relevance in the determination of food intolerance include:

1. BLOOD SUGAR FLUCTUATIONS AFTER FOOD OR CHEMICAL CHALLENGE

One of the best indications of a stress reaction in the body is a sudden rise or fall in blood sugar level, especially if this change is unrelated to a large sugar intake. An allergic reaction to a food or chemical stressor will cause such a change. The food can be a protein, carbohydrate or fat such as cheese, beef, wheat, soy milk, yeast and potato, or chemicals such as exhaust fumes, cigarette smoke and other chemical inhalants. Almost any food or chemical can cause a rapid increase in blood sugar level (hyperglycaemia) or a rapid decrease in blood sugar level (hypoglycaemia) if the person is reacting adversely to the substance. These changes are easily measured by a glucometer after a person has eaten a suspect food (or chemical). A glucometer is a machine which measures the glucose concentration in a small droplet of blood obtained by pricking the finger.

The common symptoms of hypoglycaemia — chronic fatigue, depression, anxiety, irritability, insomnia, heart palpitations, sweating, muscle pains, headaches, difficulty concentrating — are often caused by food and chemical sensitivities and not from eating too much sugar. For this reason a 3-5 hour glucose tolerance test (GTT) is often useless. It may indicate that the person is reacting adversely to a drink containing 50 grams of glucose, but this may be secondary to the food and/or chemical stressors.

The 12-hour fast which all patients undergo, just before the GTT, may in itself elicit a wide array of symptoms during the test. Many withdrawal symptoms start to arise after a 12-hour abstinence from a reactive food and may coincide with the GTT test time, causing an abnormal glucose tolerance test result and also accounting for many of the symptoms experienced during such a test.

A rapid sugar intake will most certainly cause rapid changes in blood sugar levels, but an *abnormal* glucose tolerance test tracing, most frequently reveals underlying endocrinological abnormalities caused by a wide variety of agents. Foods and chemicals are among the most notable.

2. THE PULSE TEST

Dr Arthur Coca[44] discovered that some foods may increase the pulse rate in individuals with food intolerance. The normal pulse rate variation should not exceed 16 beats/min. during the day, unless you are undergoing physical or perhaps emotional exertion. If the pulse rate suddenly rises after a meal there is a strong indication that you are reacting adversely to one of the foods in that meal. Use the following procedure to test the pulse rate.

a   The pulse should be lowest in the morning. If it is elevated you can suspect house dust. Take the pulse before rising, before eating a meal and again 30, 60 and 90 minutes after eating.

b   If the pulse is elevated after the meal (by more than 16 beats/min. above normal or greater than 84 beats/min.) the test is positive. You may be reacting adversely to some ingredient in the meal.

c   Wait until the pulse returns to your resting pulse rate before any further tests. Do not test a food if the pulse is still elevated — but you can test single foods every hour if the pulse is not elevated.

d   Refrain from smoking before testing specific foods.

e   You may not react to a single exposure if you have not eaten the test food within the preceding two weeks, and if it is a cyclic allergen.

f   Test all new foods at least twice in three days.

g   Paints, insect sprays, gas, waxes, toothpaste and other environmental chemicals may also increase your pulse rate and should be considered. Test for suspected inhalants in much the same way as for foods, by sniffing a sample.

h   Note that other factors may increase your pulse rate besides allergens. These are illness, exercise, anxiety, apprehension about the pulse test itself. Watch out for these.

i   The pulse test is too variable in very young children because of their erratic activity. Many problems can also be encountered in just finding and actually taking the pulse.

The pulse test has limited diagnostic value as not all food and chemical sensitivities necessarily manifest with an increase in the pulse rate. Watch also for post-meal changes in body temperature and blood pressure. These have similar diagnostic values to the pulse test. All physiological changes related to food and/or chemical intake are important to observe but not all occur together.

3. DROP IN URINARY ASCORBIC ACID CONCENTRATION

Acute allergic and other adverse food reactions use up body stores of vitamin C very rapidly. The highest concentration of vitamin C in the body is in the white blood cells called leukocytes. These are cells involved in the cytotoxic allergy test. They are phagocytic cells and can engulf and inactivate or destroy bacteria, virus and foreign proteins or peptides which have gained entry to the blood stream. After an acute food reaction, blood and leukocyte levels of vitamin C may drop and this drop is reflected in the urine. Urinary vitamin C levels can be measured after food or chemical challenge with the aid of C-Stix, a chemical reagent stick which can be dipped into the urine to cause a colour change indicative of the vitamin C level in the urine, which ranges from 0-40mg/dl. Measure the urine before and after the meal. A sudden drop in the ascorbic acid level may indicate an adverse food reaction. Again be careful of interpretations. There may be other explanations. All of these tests must be discussed in consultation with your nutritionally oriented practitioner.

4. SALIVA PH TEST

During an acute food reaction several physiological changes take place. The most important is an increase in the body's acidity (metabolic acidosis).[45] These changes involve not only the immune system, white blood cells, saliva and the digestive system but also target tissues of the reactive food molecules (ie joints, muscles, skin, small bowel, nervous system, etc) Such changes result in increases in inflammation, redness, swelling, oedema, etc. Researchers in the US have demonstrated that the post meal salivary pH correlated well with pH changes in the duodenum (the first part of the small bowel that joins onto the stomach and accepts digestive enzymes and bicarbonate through a tube from the pancreas).

Using a special device for measuring the acidity in the duodenum (The Heidelburg Capsule) they showed that during an adverse food or chemical reaction there was an immediate blockage in the output of pancreatic bicarbonate. About two litres of this bicarbonate normally flows daily into the duodenum after meals in order to neutralise the acid contents coming through from the stomach and also to activate the pancreatic digestive enzymes. Because the blockage in bicarbonate output has been shown to coincide with a drop in salivary pH, you can get a rough idea about your pancreatic enzymes activity and bicarbonate flow and hence, acidity in your small intestines simply by measuring your salivary pH with a special pH indicator paper with a pH range of 5.00-7.00.

The normal salivary pH is usually in the range from 6.4-6.8. Just before a meal your pH should be around 6.4 and about 30 minutes after the meal should rise to 6.8 or greater. If a reactive food is eaten during a meal (or taken singularly) the pH will drop below 6.4 instead of rising to 6.8. In severe food reactions the salivary pH can drop to below 5.00, but anywhere between 5.0-6.4 is an indication of an adverse food reaction. Such food reactions can be controlled by taking bicarbonate ½-1 hour after the meal or at the commencement of symptoms resulting from the food.

SYMPTOMS OF FOOD INTOLERANCE

Look for any of the following changes after eating a suspect food: mood changes, depression, anxiety, dread, fear, sudden fatigue, abnormal sleepiness or activity, crying fits, bad temper, muscle weakness, headaches, blurring vision, joint or muscle pains or stiffness, sudden itchiness, breathlessness, sweating, increased heart rate.

One extremely sensitive monitor of mood, emotion and the thinking process as well as motor co-ordination is handwriting. After a reactive food, marked changes can occur in handwriting and drawing. This is especially noticeable in children who may be well-behaved and writing neatly in the classroom before the lunch break, but noticeably deteriorate after lunch. This change is frequently due to an adverse food reaction that started during the lunch break. 'Glue ear' and frequent ear infections will invariably vanish after food intolerances are removed. The most common food in this case is milk (and other dairy products). Bed wetting may also suddenly stop with appropriate food eliminations.

This is by no means a full list but they can be the first indication that something is not right. We are creatures of habit and have to make careful note of such changes or we are likely to unconsciously write them off as normal.

VISIBLE SIGNS OF FOOD INTOLERANCE IN CHILDREN

The allergic face is usually puffy in appearance, especially under the eyes, which may also feature dark circles called allergic shiners and horizontal wrinkles which run from the inner corners of the eyes. Cheeks and lips are often dry and scaly, with the corners of the lips cracked. The base of the ears where they join the face may be red and cracked. Eye lashes may be wet and the ends sticking together. There may also be a horizontal crease near the end of the nose (from pushing the running nose up) and children will frequently wipe their nose with the back of their arm (called the 'allergic salute'). Pot bellies in young children will disappear when the food intolerance is removed and so will abnormal bowel movements which may alternate between diarrhoea and constipation.

Many children with grain/wheat yeast intolerance have a musty smell about them, especially from their hair, which is reminiscent of hay or fresh bread. Another sign is the rhythmic banging of the head in the pillow at night or rhythmic movement of the legs. Finally, the uncontrollable gross, clumsy, disobedient, hyperactive, problem child is usually suffering from food intolerance when other more obvious factors have been ruled out.

CHAPTER 6

SELECTION
OF A
DIET PLAN

EASY WHEAT AND DAIRY-FREE DIET PLANS

As previously discussed, many unnecessary restrictions to diet planning can arise from too narrow a view on the food family concept. Even an entire family may not pose the same problems as others. The grass family (gramineae), which includes wheat, rye, barley, oats, rice, millet, corn, bamboo shoots and sugar cane is frequently involved in adverse food reactions, while the gourd family, on the other hand, which includes rockmelon (cantaloupe), honeydew, pumpkin, cucumber, squashes (butternut pumpkin and zucchini/courgettes), chokos and watermelon, is involved less frequently. For this reason such a family of foods may be rotated on a two-day basis rather than a four or seven-day basis. This allows greater flexibility when preparing foods and allows greater control of the more suspect foods.

We have already mentioned that many single foods within a food family are often the 'bad guys', while the other members are relatively innocuous. These bad guys are the ones eaten most often. In Australia, peanuts from the legume family will elicit adverse reactions more frequently than chickpeas, lentils or alfalfa. In the US, soybean derivatives are frequent offenders. Oranges cause many more reactions than other members of the citrus family such as lemons and grapefruit.

The diet plans in this book have been designed with these observations in mind. Based on the experience of thousands of Australian patients certain foods have been eliminated entirely, while other foods have been used more frequently.

These one month diet plans are as strict as most other elimination or rotation diets but allow greater variety, as most of the families of vegetables and fruits are rotated on a two-day basis, with individual vegetables and fruits rotated less frequently. In other words every *second* day the same family of vegetables or fruit may be used, but they should be *different members of that family*. If you have a vegetable from the mustard family such as broccoli on Monday, then you can have turnips on Wednesday, cauliflower on Friday and cabbage on Sunday. Note that all of these vegetables are from the same family, but *a specific vegetable is not eaten more than once each week* even though different members of the same family are eaten on four different occasions during the week. In a similar manner, carrots, celery, parsnip and parsley (all in the carrot family) may be eaten during one week but each item usually not more than once. The frequency can be increased without ill effect, at least for vegetables. Of course if any of the vegetables or fruits are known trouble makers they should be omitted from the diet from the start. Such foods are frequently cabbage, onions, capsicum, cucumber or tomatoes.

This type of diet is especially suitable for the person with the multiple food sensitivities which change from week to week. There is far less anxiety and stress involved by starting this precalculated diet than by going through the tedious task of trying to find out which specific foods are causing the problem. In fact it is quite rare to see this type of person work out all of their specific food sensitivities as they change so frequently depending on exposure, frequency and quantity consumed. Remember the basic premise that multiple cyclic food sensitivities are simply too much of a particular food eaten too frequently.

It is for this reason that elimination diets by themselves can result in a new sensitisation to one or more of the foods in such a diet. Even though the initial suspect foods have been removed, sensitisation can occur to a newly introduced food if it is eaten daily. I have on several occasions replaced the heavier gluten containing grains with soy beans for 3-6 weeks and observed an initial improvement after two weeks, give way to a rapid deterioration by six weeks resulting from sensitisation to the soy.

This problem is easily solved by eliminating the key suspect food, *while at the same time rotating the remaining foods*. The more suspect the food family, the larger the rotation cycle.

This is my approach in the following diet plans. Each diet plan gives:

a greater variety of permitted foods

b minimal chance of new food sensitisation

c greatly reduced *total* food stressors

d total removal of the prime allergenic foods (wheat and cows milk products)

e easier compliance

All foods derived from wheat and cow's milk have been completely eliminated from the diet plans outlined in this book because these two food sources pose the greatest allergenic potential (based on clinical experience in Australia).

These foods include bread, biscuits, cakes, pastries, wheat germ, wheat bran, milk, butter, cheese, cream, yoghurt, puddings, to name just a few. Other substances completely eliminated include sugar, brewer's yeast, vegemite (marmite), alcohol, cocoa (chocolate), malt, tobacco, coffee, tea and all forms of artificial colourings, flavourings, preservatives and other food additives.

Other foods which need to be watched closely such as eggs, beef, pork, oranges, and peanuts are not used more than once, or at the most twice, every week, and in small quantities. If you know you are sensitive to any of these foods do not use them. Yeast-sensitive persons should also be careful of miso and tamari soy sauce, though these soya-based fermentation products are frequently tolerated by yeast-sensitive individuals.

PRELIMINARY MODIFIED FASTING

Before starting one of the diet plans it is preferable for adults to undertake one of the following 3-4 day modified fasts. During a fast the body briefly undergoes a cleansing and purging process. It is also a time when all allergens are withdrawn from the diet. Fasting on spring or rain water is undeniably the best way to fast but frequently meets with too much patient resistance. For this reason an additional five modified fasts are outlined. They usually accomplish the same goal with better compliance and a reduction in symptoms such as headaches, nausea and increased heart rate which may arise during the fasting period. They are less dangerous than water fasts because they still contain calories, but there is always the possibility that one of the ingredients included in the fast may be allergenic. To minimise this possibility, different foods or juices may be used each day to give a 'rotated fast' and the fasting foods are ones which have minimal allergenicity. So it is really up to you to choose the most appropriate fast, keeping in mind your daily activities (which should be kept to an absolute minimum during the four days), your propensity for low blood sugar (which may drop suddenly during any fast) and hunches about any possible reactive foods included in the fast. The following list gives the order of severity of each fast and may help you in this respect:

ORDER OF SEVERITY

1 Spring or rain water.

2 Lemon and grapefruit juice

3 Mixed juice (carrot, beetroot, grapefruit, lemon, pineapple, watermelon)

4 Watermelon

5 Mixed fruit (pawpaw, rockmelon, watermelon)

6 Rice and vegetables (vegetable soup)

Those who feel they need to keep up their blood sugar level or who have had severe reactions (such as headaches) while on a previous fast, should consider fasts 3-6. If watermelons are in season try fast 4 – an excellent way to reduce fluid buildup in ankles, stomach or face. The mixed juice or fruit fasts Nos 3, 4 and 5 are best for the hot weather, and the rice and vegetables fast 6 is a good choice for the colder months of the year.

✳ Children should not fast unless under medical supervision and in a controlled environment. Start them straight into one of the diet plans. Infants 6-12 months can usually eat what the rest of the family eats but may need the food blended or mashed.

The best day to start your fast is either Thursday or Friday morning depending upon whether you are planning to go three or four days. This way by Monday morning you will be ready to start one of the diet plans and will have had the weekend to finish off the fast in case you feel particularly weak and not very mentally coherent. It is better to feel this way at home where you can relax than at work where a job has to be performed.

During the fast there are no restrictions on the amount consumed, but you may need to dilute juices further with water if your liquid consumption is too high. If you wish to start a four-day fast instead of a three-day fast, use Sunday's outline on Thursday. Now choose one of the six suggested fasts making sure to eat or drink only the suggested foods or juices. If you have to break a fast for any reason do it gently by eating moderate amounts of vegetables, grains, fruit and fish, rather than sugar, fat, refined foods or meat.

FRIDAY

Fast No. 1 Spring *or* rain water (unlimited quantity)

Fast No. 2 Lemon juice 1½ cups in 2 litres (or more) (unlimited)

Fast No. 3 Lemon and/or grapefruit 1½-2 cups mixed in 2 litres or more of water (unlimited)

Fast No. 4 Watermelon (unlimited)

Fast No. 5 Fresh paw paw (papaya) *or* pears (unlimited) and water unlimited

Fast No. 6 Rice & vegetable soup (use different types of vegetables each day)

SATURDAY

Fast No. 1 Spring *or* rain water (unlimited quantity)

Fast No. 2 Grapefruit juice 700 mls in 2 litres water (or more) (unlimited)

Fast No. 3 Fresh raw beetroot (beet) juice & fresh raw carrot juice (mixed together 1:1 or alternating) all juice mixed 50% with water (unlimited)

Fast No. 4 Watermelon (unlimited)

Fast No. 5 Fresh rockmelon (unlimited) and water unlimited

Fast No. 6   Vegetable soup (use different types of vegetables each day)

SUNDAY (and Thursday if 4 day fast)

Fast No. 1   Spring or rain water (unlimited quantity)

Fast No. 2   Lemon juice 1½ cups in 2 litres water (or more) (unlimited)

Fast No. 3   Fresh ripe pineapple diluted 50% with water (2 litres) and pieces of watermelon (unlimited) but not eaten at the same time as the pineapple.

Fast No. 4   Watermelon (unlimited)

Fast No. 5   Watermelon (unlimited) *or* paw paw (papaya) and water (unlimited)

Fast No. 6   Rice and vegetable soup (use different types of vegetables each day)

STARTING ONE OF THE DIET PLANS

If you have just completed one of the 3-4 day fasts (which is recommended but not an absolute prerequisite), now choose one of the diet plans and make sure you keep your overall food intake low during the next few days. Gradually increase your food consumption and avoid overeating. Let your body slowly get used to an increased food load.

During the fast period you may have unmasked a hidden food sensitivity. When you eat this food again it may cause symptoms such as headaches, wheezing, stuffy nose, difficulty breathing, stomach pains, diarrhoea, behaviour and mood changes and so on. Watch for such changes and record any symptoms experienced during this first week. You can then correlate them with the meal eaten before the symptoms started.

Some people have found that by eating just one type of food as a meal, during the first week they can more accurately relate signs and symptoms with a specific allergenic food (eg pumpkin for breakfast, fish for lunch, bananas for dinner, potatoes for breakfast). Having pinpointed the offending foods in this manner they can then be completely eliminated from the diet.

However, such a procedure is not necessary for those with cyclic food sensitivities and especially those with multiple food intolerance because the adverse reactions associated with these reactive foods can be adequately controlled by reducing the quantity and frequency of consumption of the specific food. Remember that the major allergenic foods (wheat and milk) have already been removed and will be introduced later in a predetermined manner, and you have already eliminated any foods which are consistent trouble makers. The remaining foods are more likely to be tolerated with spacing.

If, however, you do get an acute reaction after one meal, test each component in that meal again by itself during the following week. If you still get acute reactions remove it from your diet.

By using the single food as a meal approach it is indeed possible to locate the potential trouble maker but such a trouble maker which also has the potential for causing chronic degenerative disease if repeatedly consumed in quantity may not be a trouble maker if consumed every 4-7 days in smaller quantities.

For this reason we are not testing foods as single meals after the fast, but making the assumption that the foods causing fixed allergies have already been eliminated. Knowing exactly which of the remaining foods are cyclic allergens is not important, as they are constantly changing according to exposure and stress levels of the individual. What is more important is to relieve the body immediately of all potential or present cyclic food sensitivies by rotating all foods in the diet, because they are constantly changing, so the bad guy today may not necessarily be the bad guy tomorrow. This approach also completely eliminates the possibility of a gradual build up of a specific food sensitivity as no foods are eaten more than twice each week (with one or two exceptions).

Several diet plans are available, some for cold weather, some for hot weather and others for mid season. Some are simple, some more complex and one is included for the vegetarian.

The four-day rotation Rice Diet Plan no. 13 does not rotate the whole grain brown rice, but rather emphasises its use at nearly every meal. The justification for this is based purely on clinical experience. If the patient does not have a rice sensitivity (and it is rare to build up such a sensitivity in four weeks) I know of no better food for losing excess weight quickly, correcting hormone imbalances, reducing fluid build up, normalising bowel movements, stabilising blood sugar levels and inducing a calm, centred and less emotional state, while at the same time supplying a staple food largely free of gluten and high in vitamins, minerals and good quality fibre. Two additional four-day rotation diet plans (nos 7 & 8) rotate rice every two days. Use rice which has been organically grown and free of chemical sprays.

When you have completed four weeks on your selected diet plan (or even longer if you are doing well and enjoying it) you can start to modify your diet by including other meals suggested in the Wheat and Dairy Free Recipes section. At this stage you should be able to cope with a greater variety of foods, perhaps rotated less frequently. You may even like to rotate the meats or vegetables in the diet plan in a different order during weeks 2, 3 and 4, but keep an eye on the individual food spacing. Keep the same rotation frequency.

CONTROL OF FOOD PREPARATION AND PURCHASING

You will find it much easier, at least for the first 3-4 weeks if you eat all meals at home or make prior arrangements concerning food if eating out. It may be easier for the first month of the new diet program for you to organise social activities around your own home. In this way you control the food selection at dinner parties, morning and afternoon snacks etc. Organise a picnic or barbeque where you again control the food preparation, at least for your family. Encourage neighbouring children to play at your house so you prepare the snacks for the children. If you have to eat out try to select a suitable restaurant which serves a selection of fresh whole foods you can eat. Don't be afraid to ask the waiter what is in each food. Ask for sauces to be served on the side rather than flowing over the food. You can always ask for fresh fruit for dessert, for example strawberries without cream or icecream. Spend your time with friends who are likely to understand what you are endeavouring to do. If you are invited out to dinner, offer to bring a plate of food, or invite them to your place instead.

It is especially important that you control the food situation during the first month of the program.

When shopping always read the labels to make sure all ingredients are acceptable to your specific diet, but remember that many hidden additives are not always mentioned and frequently include corn, wheat, dairy products, egg, soy and yeast. For this reason it is advisable to choose *only* whole unprocessed foods including fruit, vegetables, whole grains, legumes, fish and lamb which have not gone through any manufacturing process. If possible, get your food 'spray free' and try to buy seasonal produce. Do not rely on cans and packets.

Initially this may appear to be a more expensive way of shopping. Obviously it is less expensive to live on bread, sausages and spaghetti. This diet, however, has the advantage of completely eliminating many foods such as wheat products (cakes, pastries, bread), dairy products (ice cream, cheesecakes, fancy cheeses), alcoholic beverages, coffee, condiments and of course, cigarettes. Such changes cut down on the food bill significantly. If whole grains and vegetables are used as staples and selected cuts of meats and fish are chosen with an eye on economy, the *total* weekly food bill may not necessarily be more expensive than before. In the long run the improvement in health may considerably reduce the cost of health care such as doctors' bills, hospitals, and medication.

It is preferable to seek out a source of cheaper bulk dry foods such as grains and legumes, but do not purchase bulk quantities of fresh foods. You may buy what you need for a week but this would mean purchasing fewer foods of a greater variety. Where you may have been purchasing a 5kg (10lb) bag of oranges and apples, you may now need to buy 4 apples, 4 oranges, 4 bananas, 4 pears, a rockmelon/cantaloupe, a pawpaw/papaya, a piece of watermelon and some berries. The limitation to quantity will depend on how long each food will keep. Freshness is important. It is usually possible to rotate easily perishable fruits and vegetables in the first part of the week while others remain fresh in the refrigerator or are still coming to complete ripeness.

Some meals you may prepare in bulk. Freeze two portions while eating the third. This saves cooking time. The frozen portions should be well marked for future use in your rotation diet. Another time saver and an economical procedure for using up 'left overs' involves taking meat surplus from dinner for lunches the next day (see Diet Plan No. 2). In this way the rotated meat of the day is consumed within a 24-hour period, but the period is from evening to evening instead of breakfast to breakfast. A minority will find that they need the 12-hour fast during the night to separate each rotated food but the majority will find that the flow through of a specific food from dinner to lunch the next day a much more economical and realistic approach and this leads to better compliance in the long run.

Don't forget to use time saving appliances such as the crockpot and pressure cooker. The crockpot is an excellent time saver when cooking grains, legumes and meat dishes. Enough brown rice for a week can be cooked in a pressure cooker and stored in the refrigerator in a sealed container for use in puddings, cereals, fried rice and rice salads. Similarly stewed fruit will keep in the refrigerator while fresh fruit may not last to the second rotated day.

CHAPTER 7

DIET
PLANS AND
RECIPES

Recipes for the Diet Plans can be found later in this chapter.

DIET PLANS

1 Simple Diet No. 1   72
2 Simple Diet No. 2   74
3 Summer Diet   75
4 Autumn Diet   78
5 Winter Diet   80
6 Spring Diet   82
7 Two Day Rice Rotation No. 1   86
8 Two Day Rice Rotation No. 2   87
9 Toddlers Diet   88
10 School Lunch Ideas   89
11 Infants Diet 6-12 months   91
12 Vegetarian Diet   92
13 Rice Diet   94

1- 6   Diet Plans are seven day rotation diets
7-12   Diet Plans are four day rotation diets

SIMPLE SEVEN DAY ROTATION DIET PLAN No. 1
Monday
Breakfast   Grapefruit *or* pears. Eggs.
Lunch   Avocado/Seafood salad *or* Corn on the cob.

Dinner   Baked Chicken. Peas, beans, carrots, parsnips. Apricots with Almond Cream.

Snacks   Almonds, popcorn, pears.

Tuesday

Breakfast   Lemon juice. Millet porridge with dates and cashew milk.

Lunch   Fried Rice *or* Salmon Rissoles.

Dinner   Baked Fish. Rice. Zucchini/courgettes, sweet potato. Watermelon.

Snacks   Ricecakes, dates, olives, pumpkin seeds.

Wednesday

Breakfast   Peaches *or* banana. Oats *or* barley cereal with raisins. Soy milk.

Lunch   100% rye bread sandwich with ham, sprouts and grated carrot.

Dinner   Lamb chops. Carrots, parsnips, beets, Brussels sprouts. Mandarin.

Snacks   Chips (potato), pine nuts, Brazil nuts, carrot juice.

Thursday

Breakfast   Lemon and honey drink. Sago with stewed prunes and almond milk.

Lunch   Prawn/shrimp rice salad (celery, parsley, leeks, tomato, lettuce/Webb's wonder/iceberg).

Dinner   Rockmelon/cantaloupe slice. Mediterranean style mullet (or other fish). Fried eggplant/aubergine.

Snacks   Almonds, apples, paw paw/papaya.

Friday

Breakfast   Pineapple *or* mango. Eggs.

Lunch   Corn on the cob *or* fruit salad (pear, fig, watermelon, mango, banana, pineapple).

Dinner   Steamed Chicken. Sweet potato, cauliflower, broccoli, corn. Banana split (cashew cream).

Snacks   Watermelon, popcorn, bananas, pistachio nuts.

Saturday

Breakfast Oranges *or* paw paw/papaya. Barley cereal with soy *or* goats milk.

Lunch Potato salad (garlic, radish, cucumber, sprouts, zucchini/courgettes, with sardines.

Dinner Baked Fish (ginger, garlic, tamari). Chinese vegetables. Fresh berries.

Snacks Sunflower seeds, pine nuts, peaches, paw paw/papaya.

Sunday

Breakfast Brown rice with raisins and cashew milk.

Lunch Barbecued veal *or* beef. Fried onions. Rice salad. Bunch of grapes.

Dinner Pork chops with apple sauce. Salad (lettuce/Webb's wonder/iceberg, tomato, capsicum/red or green pepper, onion, celery). Kiwi fruit/gooseberries *or* plums.

Snacks Olives, pistachio nuts, pumpkin seeds, sultanas/seedless raisins, rice cakes.

SIMPLE DIET   DIET PLAN No. 2

Monday

Breakfast Bacon, tomato. Banana.

Lunch Tuna and rice. Alfalfa sprouts.

Dinner Prawns/shrimps, scallops. Rice and tomato.

Tuesday

Breakfast Rice (boiled). Stewed Apple. Almond milk. Currants.

Lunch Salmon, asparagus, corn. Apple.

Dinner Omelette, corn, parsley.

Wednesday

Breakfast Scrambled eggs. 100% rye bread. Fresh grapes.

Lunch Hard-boiled egg. Beetroot/beet and celery.

Dinner Chicken. Carrots, zucchini/courgettes and spinach/spring or collard greens.

Thursday

Breakfast Paw paw/papaya *or* melon.

Lunch Chicken leg *or* breast. Pineapple.

Dinner Lamb. Pumpkin and green beans.

Friday

Breakfast Lambs fry/liver *and/or* fried onions and mushrooms. Fresh pineapple.

Lunch Cold lamb chop/chump or rib chop. Salad. (tomato and corn).

Dinner Fish. Lemon rice and broccoli.

Saturday

Breakfast Kippers with lemon. One fresh grapefruit.

Lunch Lentil beef soup. Sprout salad with walnuts and cucumber.

Dinner Roast beef *or* steak, potato and peas.

Sunday

Breakfast Goats yogurt or pears.

Lunch Cold roast beef. Lettuce/Webb's wonder/iceberg, radish, with French dressing.

Dinner Pork, cauliflower and sweet potato.

During this diet plan, single foods are consumed once only during any 24 hour period. This is an example of a simple 7 day rotation diet. Modify this one to suit your own needs.

SEVEN DAY ROTATION DIET PLAN No. 3 SUMMER

Monday

Breakfast Paw paw/papaya *or* rockmelon/cantaloupe. Cornbread with almond butter.

Lunch Corn on the cob. Chicken *or* egg. Salad with grated carrot and beetroot/beet.

Dinner Chicken soup *or* oysters. Prawn/shrimp avocado salad. Fruit salad with tahini/sesame seed paste.

Snacks Pop corn, corn chips, advocado dip, pecan nuts, hummus.

Cooking suggestions Salad dressing: tahini, honey and grapefruit, corn oil and honey. Almond milk, almond oil, sesame oil, tahini, kudzu (thickener).

Tuesday

Breakfast Mango slices *or* fresh berries with cashew cream.

Lunch Fish fillets. Rice salad with pineapple and seeds.

Dinner Paul's Favourite Tuna Dish. Watermelon.

Snacks Pistachio nuts, pumpkin seeds, rice cakes, rice crackers, dates, watermelon.

Cooking suggestions Salad dressing: olive oil and lemon, safflower oil and lemon. Agar, arrowroot, rice vinegar, rice syrups.

Wednesday

Breakfast Homemade Muesli with soy banana milk *or* yogurt.

Lunch Rye bread sandwich: ham *or* tomato, or lentil purée.

Dinner Lamb chops. Buckwheat noodles with garlic and tomato sauce. Tofu *or* banana whip.

Snacks Hot chips (potato), crisp chips, pine nuts, Brazil nuts. Beet *or* carrot juice.

Cooking suggestions Salad dressing: peanut oil, soy sauce and vinegar. Peanut oil, gelatin, carob, black sugar, vinegar, soy milk, tamari. Use 100% rye bread (yeast free).

Thursday

Breakfast Lemon sago with grated apple *or* millet cereal with stewed apple and almond milk.

Lunch Rice salad with crab *or* prawns/shrimp. Half rockmelon/cantaloupe.

Dinner Steamed calamari. Taboulie (Lebanese green salad) with millet. Kiwi fruit jelly/gooseberry jelly/gelatin *or* apple-rhubarb crumble.

Snacks Rice cakes. Slice of paw pay/papaya *or* rockmelon/cantaloupe.

Cooking suggestions Salad dressing: lemon, tahini and honey *or* avocado and lemon. Almond milk, almond oil, agar, kudzu (thickener), sago, honey, rice syrup.

Friday

Breakfast   Fresh pineapple juice *or* mango slices. Eggs *or* corn on the cob.

Lunch   Large fruit salad with cashew cream (pear, fig, watermelon, mango, pineapple, banana).

Dinner   Chicken pieces baked in pineapple juice. Green salad with broccoli and mustard cress. Banana split with cashew cream and pistachio nuts.

Snacks   Green drink. Watermelon, bananas, popcorn, corn chips.

Cooking suggestions   Corn oil, arrowroot, tapioca flour, molasses.

Saturday

Breakfast   Fresh orange juice. Homemade muesli *or* paw paw/papaya.

Lunch   Potato salad (including sprouts, cucumber, zucchini/courgettes, with beetroot/beet). Rockmelon/cantaloupe balls.

Dinner   Japanese stir-fried fish with Chinese cabbage and sprouts. Fresh berries.

Snacks   Roasted sunflower seeds, pine nuts, macadamia nuts.

Cooking suggestions   Soy milk, soy oil, sunflower oil, safflower oil, tamari, agar, carob, coconut, maple syrup, golden syrup/light corn syrup.

Sunday

Breakfast   Fresh grape juice. Apple sunrise with yogurt (if allowed). Fried eggplant/aubergine.

Lunch   Barbecued beef kebabs *or* wheat free veal sausages. Waldorf salad. Watermelon.

Dinner   Stuffed tomato (olives, celery, capsicum/red or green pepper, parsley). Family Fried Rice (onion, bacon, pumpkin seeds, capsicum, chili). Bunch of grapes *or* mango sherbet.

Snacks   Grapes, watermelon, olives, ricecakes, pistachio nuts, pumpkin seeds, sultanas.

Cooking suggestions   Salad dressing: olive oil with cider vinegar or olive oil with wine vinegar. Rice syrup, gelatin, grape seed oil.

SEVEN DAY ROTATION DIET PLAN No. 4   AUTUMN/FALL

Monday

Breakfast   Fresh pears. Scrambled eggs with sprouts. Cornbread.

Lunch   Corn salad with leeks, beets, radish, cucumber *or* avocado and seafood.

Dinner   Dal. Chicken curry. Fruit salad and tahini.

Snacks   Hummus with corn chips, almonds, avocado dip, popcorn, pecan nuts.

Cooking suggestions   Salad dressing: tahini and grapefruit. Almond milk, almond oil, sesame oil, corn oil, honey, kudzu (thickener).

Tuesday

Breakfast   Millet and linseed cereal with dates and cashew milk. Potato pancakes/crepes.

Lunch   Fried rice.

Dinner   Stir-fry fish and vegetables with rice. Pineapple jelly/gelatin *or* sweet potato sorbet.

Snacks   Olives, pistachio nuts, pumpkin seeds, rice cakes, dates.

Cooking suggestions   Salad dressing: olive oil and lemon, safflower oil and lemon. Agar, arrowroot, rice vinegar, rice syrup.

Wednesday

Breakfast   Stewed pears with yogurt *or* tofu, banana and fig cream. Lambs fry/liver.

Lunch   100% rye bread sandwich: 1) ham and salad 2) soy and lentil spread.

Dinner   Split pea and ham soup. Lamb and tomato kebabs. Apricot sorbet.

Snacks   Mandarin, hot chips, crisp chips, pine nuts, Brazil nuts, carrot juice.

Cooking suggestions   Peanut oil, gelatin, carob, black sugar, vinegar, soy milk, tamari.

Thursday

Breakfast   Prune juice. Millet *or* sago cereal with stewed apple.

Lunch   Millet casserole *or* prawn/shrimp rice salad *or* calamari salad.

Dinner Half a rockmelon/cantaloupe. Seafood kebabs *or* Mediter-ranean style mullet, Baked apple.

Snacks Pop corn.

Cooking suggestions Salad dressing: lemon and tahini and honey. Almond milk, almond oil, agar, kudzu (thickener), sage, honey, rice syrup.

Friday

Breakfast Fresh pineapple juice. Eggs *or* buckwheat pancake/crepe.

Lunch Corn pones. Carrot and currant salad.

Dinner Steamed chicken. Carrots, sweet potato, broccoli, okra. Stewed quinces.

Snacks Green drink, watermelon, bananas, dried bananas, corn chips, pop corn.

Cooking suggestions Corn oil, arrowroot, tapioca flour, molasses.

Saturday

Breakfast Fresh orange juice. Barley cereal with soy *or* goats milk.

Lunch Potato salad with soy mayonnaise, pine nuts, garlic, radish, cucumber garnished with sardines or anchovies. Marinated mushrooms.

Dinner Fish curry with coconut milk. Cucumber (and yogurt). Potato sambal. Compote of fresh berries.

Snacks Oranges, dried paw paw/papaya, pine nuts, macadamia nuts, roasted sunflower seeds.

Cooking suggestions Soy milk, soy oil, sunflower oil, safflower oil, tamari, agar, carob, coconut, maple syrup, golden syrup/light corn syrup.

Sunday

Breakfast Stewed prunes with goats yogurt (optional). Thickened apples (tapioca flour).

Lunch Barbecued beef, veal, pork, with fried rice and mashed pumpkin with nutmeg.

Dinner Pork chops with apple sauce *or* Chili Con Carne. Salad (lettuce/Webb's wonder/iceberg, tomato, capsicum,) and celery.

Snacks Olives, kiwi fruit/gooseberries, pistachio nuts, sultanas/seedless raisins, rice cakes.

Cooking suggestions Olive oil, rice syrup, gelatin, grape seed oil.

SEVEN DAY ROTATION DIET PLAN No. 5 WINTER

Monday

Breakfast Grapefruit juice. Eggs. Chicken sausage (wheat free). Cornbread with almond butter.

Lunch Winter salad – grated parsnips, beets, radish, cucumber with bean dressing.

Dinner Borscht soup. Baked chicken with peas, beans, carrots, parsnips. Baked pears with almond cream.

Snacks Pop corn, corn chips, avocado dip, hummus, figs, almonds, dried pears, paw paw/papaya.

Cooking suggestions Salad dressing: pinto beans, tahini and grapefruit. Almond milk, almond oil, sesame oil, corn oil, honey, kudzu (thickener).

Tuesday

Breakfast Lemon juice. Millet and linseed cereal with cashew milk. Smoked kippers.

Lunch Winter salad – grated pumpkin, onion, celery, turnip, zucchini/courgettes *or* fried rice.

Dinner Pumpkin soup. Baked fish. Rice. Zucchini/courgettes, sweet potato, broccoli. Lemon jelly/gelatin.

Snacks Pistachio nuts, pumpkin seeds, rice cakes, dates, olives.

Cooking suggestions Salad dressing: olive oil with lemon juice *or* safflower oil with lemon juice. Agar, arrowroot, rice vinegar, rice syrup.

Wednesday

Breakfast Oats *or* barley cereal with soy milk *or* yogurt and figs and raisins. Potato cakes/fritters.

Lunch Split pea and ham soup. 100% rye bread sandwich *or* Lentil stew.

Dinner   Roast lamb with garlic slivers. Carrots, parsnips, beets, Brussels sprouts. Tofu and fig whip *or* mandarin segments.

Snacks   Mandarin, potato chips, pine nuts, Brazil nuts, carrot juice.

Cooking suggestions   Peanut oil, gelatin, carob, black sugar, vinegar, soy milk, tamari.

Thursday

Breakfast   Lemon and honey drink. Millet cereal with stewed prunes and almond milk.

Lunch   Leftover lamb. Millet casserole.

Dinner   Fried fresh anchovies *or* sardines. Ratatouille. Fruit and nut crumble.

Snacks   Apples, almonds, dried paw paw/papaya.

Cooking suggestions   Almond milk, almond oil, agar, kudzu (thickener), sago, honey, rice syrup. Salad dressing: lemon with tahini and honey.

Friday

Breakfast   Half a grapefruit. Tapioca with figs. Scrambled eggs with sprouts *or* buckwheat pancake/crepe.

Lunch   Chicken livers *or* hard-boiled egg *or* omelette. Carrot and currant salad.

Dinner   Steamed chicken. Sweet potato, cauliflower and broccoli. Figs stewed in pineapple juice with cashew cream.

Snacks   Dried paw paw/papaya. Fresh paw paw/papaya. Currants, pistachio nuts, dried banana.

Cooking suggestions   Corn oil, arrowroot, tapioca flour, molasses.

Saturday

Breakfast   Fresh orange juice. Roasted barley cereal with soy *or* date milk. Grilled fish.

Lunch   Lentil soup. Potato pancakes/crepes *or* winter salad (radish, cabbage, parsnips, sprouts).

Dinner   Mushroom and barley soup. Baked fish with fried parsnips and sautéed zucchini/courgettes.

Snacks   Oranges, pine nuts, macadamia nuts, roasted sunflower seeds.

Cooking suggestions   Soy milk, soy oil, sunflower oil, safflower oil, tamari, agar, carob, coconut, maple syrup, golden syrup/light corn syrup.

Sunday

Breakfast   Fresh apple juice. Rice cereal with raisins and cashew milk *or* veal sausages and grilled tomato.

Lunch   Barbecued veal *or* pork with tangy rice salad *or* steak and kidney pie. Green salad (lettuce *or* spinach).

Dinner   Beef casserole (tomato, capsicum/red or green pepper, eggplant/aubergine, olives, celery). Boiled rice. Hot fruit salad with cashew cream (raisins, currants, sultanas/seedless raisins, prunes, apple).

Snacks   Olives, raisins, currants, prunes.

Cooking suggestions   Grape seed oil, olive oil. Salad dressing: olive oil with cider vinegar *or* olive oil with wine vinegar. Rice syrup, gelatin.

SEVEN DAY ROTATION DIET PLAN No. 6   SPRING

Monday

Breakfast   Fresh grapefruit juice. Scrambled eggs with papadams *or* chopped popcorn with almond milk.

Lunch   Chick pea salad *or* avocado and seafood.

Dinner   Fresh asparagus *or* artichoke. Chicken pieces baked in apricot nectar. Carob gelato.

Snacks   Almonds, pecans, dried pears, popcorn, hummus with corn chips.

Cooking suggestions   Almond milk, almond oil, sesame oil, corn oil, honey, kudzu (thickener).

Tuesday

Breakfast   Millet and linseed cereal with cashew milk.

Lunch   Cauliflower with mint salad *or* salmon rissoles with pumpkin.

Dinner   Fish curry with coconut cream. Rice. Stewed cherry jelly/gelatin.

Snacks Pistachio nuts, pumpkin seeds, rice cakes, dates, olives.

Cooking suggestions Salad dressing: olive oil with lemon, *or* safflower oil with lemon. Agar, arrowroot, rice vinegar, rice syrup.

Wednesday

Breakfast Peaches and banana with yogurt (if allowed). Eggless potato pancake/crepe.

Lunch 100% rye bread sandwich, ham salad *or* lentil purée.

Dinner Rack of lamb with fried parsnips and spring vegetables. Tofu or peach whip.

Snacks Hot potato chips, or crisp chips, pine nuts, Brazil nuts, carrot juice.

Cooking suggestions Peanut oil, gelatin, carob, black sugar, vinegar, soy milk, tamari.

Thursday

Breakfast Lemon *or* honey drink. Millet *or* sago with stewed apple. Almond milk.

Lunch Marinated calamari or avocado and mussel salad *or* lamb (leftover) salad.

Dinner Sautéed scallops *or* fried anchovies. Ratatouille. Apple crumble.

Snacks Almonds, apples, pawpaw/papaya.

Cooking suggestions Almond milk, almond oil, agar, kudzu (thickener), sago, honey, rice syrup. Salad dressing: lemon with tahini and honey.

Friday

Breakfast Fresh pineapple juice *or* mango slices. Eggs.

Lunch Corn on the cob *or* large fruit salad (pear, fig, watermelon, mango, pineapple, banana) with cashew cream.

Dinner Chicken pieces baked in pineapple juice. Steamed broccoli. Banana split with cashew cream and pistachios.

Snacks Pistachio nuts, Green drink, watermelon, bananas, popcorn, cornchips.

Cooking suggestions Corn oil, arrowroot, tapioca flour, molasses.

Saturday

Breakfast Fresh orange juice. Paw paw/papaya. Fish rissoles.

Lunch Kidney beans (garlic, mushrooms and soy sauce) on toast. 100% rye bread. Peaches *or* fresh lychee nuts.

Dinner Steamed *or* baked fish (garlic, ginger, tamari). Chinese vegetables. Creamed strawberry tofu.

Snacks Pine nuts, macadamia nuts, sunflower seeds, peaches, oranges, paw paw/papaya, strawberries.

Cooking suggestions Soy milk, soy oil, sunflower, safflower oils, tamari, agar, carob, coconut, maple syrup, golden syrup/light corn syrup.

Sunday

Breakfast Brown rice (hot or cold) with grated apple, walnuts, Brazil nuts. Cashew cream *or* yogurt. Grilled bacon and tomato.

Lunch Barbecued beef, veal or pork. Salad (spinach, lettuce, olives, capsicum/red or green pepper, celery, onion, parsley. Plums in season.

Dinner Spinach pie. Baked apples with sultanas/seedless raisins, walnuts and rice syrup.

Snacks Olives, pistachio nuts, pumpkin seeds, sultanas/seedless raisins, rice cakes.

Cooking suggestions Salad dressing: olive oil with cider vinegar *or* olive oil with wine vinegar. Olive oil, rice syrup. Gelatin, grape seed oil.

FOUR DAY ROTATION DIETARY FOOD SELECTION   TO BE USED FOR DIET PLANS Nos 7-10

- Incorporates rice every two days
- Also see the following two diet plans

Day 1

Animal proteins Squid, crab, mussels, clams. Chicken, chicken livers. Eggs. Rabbit.

Vegetable proteins Chick peas/garbanzos, pinto beans, black beans, lentils. Sesame, walnuts.

Vegetables   Alfalfa sprouts, lentil sprouts, celery, parsley, pumpkin, zucchini/courgettes, artichoke, chicory/French or Belgian endive, lettuce/Webb's wonder/iceberg.

Grains and substitutes   Corn, millet, rice, rye.

Fruits   Honeydew melon, watermelon, custard apple, pineapple, gooseberries/kiwifruit.

Snacks   Rice cakes, pop corn, dried pineapple, nuts and fruit as above.

Cooking suggestions   Cornmeal, rice flour, sesame oil, safflower oil, tahini, black sugar, golden syrup/light corn syrup, agar, camomile tea, corn syrup, rice syrup, molasses, rice noodles.

Day 2

Animal proteins   Flounder, snapper/sea bass, bream, sole, herring, jewfish. Duck. Beef, veal, liver, kidney.

Vegetable proteins   Cashew, pistachio, pine nuts.

Vegetables   Broccoli, horseradish, mustard greens, radish, turnip, tomato, chili, capsicum/red or green pepper, eggplant/ aubergine, onion, shallots, beetroot/beet, capers, olives.

Grains and substitutes   Sago.

Fruits   Mango, grapefruit, lemon, tangerine, mandarin, pear, quince, peach, plum, raspberries, blackberries, dates.

Snacks   Prunes. Nuts and fruit as above.

Cooking suggestions   Olive oil, date sugar, gelatine, rosehip tea, basil, oregano, cayenne, black pepper, bay leaves, cloves.

Day 3

Animal proteins   Oysters, abalone, scallops, lobster, prawns/shrimp. Turkey. Pork, ham, bacon.

Vegetable proteins   Split peas, soy beans, kidney beans. Peanuts, pecans, sunflower seeds.

Vegetables   Peas, stringbeans, mung bean sprouts, carrot, parsnip, cucumber, squash/marrow, sweet potato, dandelion greens, endive/chicory, mushrooms, bamboo shoots, water chestnuts.

Grains and substitutes   Rice, arrowroot.

Fruits Rockmelon/cantaloupe, grapes, paw paw/papaya, banana, mulberry, fig, blueberry.

Snacks Rice cakes. Nut and fruits as above.

Cooking suggestions Rice flour, carob, wine vinegar, soy oil, sunflower oil, peanut oil, ginger, turmeric, honey, lemongrass tea, lecithin, kelp, tamari, rice noodles.

Day 4

Animal proteins Sardines, salmon, tuna, anchovy, flathead, gemfish, mullet, whitebait. Quail, pheasant and their eggs. Lamb brains.

Vegetable proteins Almonds, Brazil nuts.

Vegetables Brussels sprouts, cabbage, swede/rutabaga, cauliflower, watercress, mint, potato, asparagus, chives, garlic, leek, spinach, avocado.

Grains and substitutes Buckwheat, tapioca.

Fruits Lime, orange, rhubarb, apple, apricot, cherry, strawberries, coconut, lychees.

Snacks Nuts and fruits as above.

Cooking suggestions Potato flour, coconut oil, coconut milk, maple syrup, rosemary, white pepper, cinnamon, allspice, 100% buckwheat noodles.

Using this dietary selection table you can make up your own diet plan menus similar to the two that follow.

FOUR DAY ROTATION DIET PLAN No. 7
• Incorporates rice every two days.

Day 1

Breakfast Honeydew melon or watermelon. Eggs.

Lunch Sautéed chicken livers or chicken and lentil salad (alfalfa, celery, parsley lettuce/Webb's wonder/Iceberg)

Dinner Mussel soup. Large fried rice with chicken, celery, parsley. Pineapple jelly/gelatin.

Day 2

Breakfast Prunes (soaked or stewed). Grilled fillet of bream/sea bass/porgy.

Lunch Sautéed beef kidneys. Raw salad of broccoli, grated radish and turnip, shallots, mustard greens.

Dinner Veal chops. Ratatouille (Italian style). Lemon sago.

Day 3

Breakfast Paw paw/papaya, topped with banana, sunflower seeds, pecan nuts.

Lunch Oriental bean salad. Brown rice.

Dinner Baked turkey breast with brown rice and sautéed mushrooms. Squash/marrow/winter squash and peas. Mulberries or grapes.

Day 4

Breakfast Apricots, strawberries or grated apple. Deep fried whitebait (rolled in potato flour).

Lunch Avocado *or* salmon potato rissoles. Watercress or cabbage salad. Salad dressing: lime juice, almond oil, chives, and garlic.

Dinner Roast lamb with rosemary. Baked potato and swede/rutabaga and spinach. Fresh lychee *or* baked apple with almond cream.

FOUR DAY ROTATION DIET PLAN No. 8

• Incorporates rice every two days

Day 1

Breakfast Fresh pineapple. Corn bread.

Lunch Crab and rice salad (celery, parsley, raw zucchini/courgettes, lettuce/Webb's wonder/iceberg, toasted sesame seeds).

Dinner Baked chicken with pumpkin, rice, zucchini/courgettes, artichoke hearts. Kiwifruit/gooseberries or melon.

Day 2

Breakfast Half grapefruit. Poached herring.

Lunch Lambs fry/liver (if desired). Raw salad (see vegetable choice in dietary selection table). Salad dressing: lemon juice, olive oil, basil.

Dinner Borscht soup. Steak and kidney with grilled tomato and broccoli. Baked pear with cashew cream.

Day 3

Breakfast Hot brown rice with currants. Soy milk with banana, fig and honey.

Lunch Prawn/shrimp fried rice (peas, mung bean sprouts, carrot, mushroom, bamboo shoots, water chestnuts).

Dinner Prosciutto melon. Roast pork. Toasted sunflower rice, fried parsnips and green beans. Pecans and muscatel grapes.

Day 4

Breakfast Grated apple with orange juice, coconut and almond cream. Lamb brains.

Lunch Half an avocado. Potato salad with mint, chives and watercress. Salad dressing: lime juice, almond oil, garlic, chives.

Dinner Grilled *or* barbecued mullet (or other fish listed). Fresh asparagus with lime juice. Stewed apple and rhubarb *or* fresh apricots *or* cherries.

FOUR DAY ROTATION DIET PLAN No. 9 TODDLERS

Day 1

Breakfast Egg yolk with fingers of 100% rye toast. Custard apple.

Lunch Celery sticks with hummus. Corn on the cob (blended for very young children). Watermelon.

Dinner Steamed chicken. Pumpkin. Lettuce/Webb's wonder/iceberg, and parsley salad. Pineapple jelly/gelatin.

Drinks and snacks Water*. Diluted fresh pineapple juice. Rice cakes with tahini *or* hummus.

* Whenever possible children should be encouraged to drink water. Fruit juice should be used as a treat eg. at breakfast when vitamins might be difficult to swallow.

Day 2

Breakfast Stewed prunes and sago with cashew milk. Fish if desired.

Lunch Tomato slices with puréed cooked eggplant/aubergine, olive oil, onion *or* fish fillet with tomato. Mandarin.

Dinner Beetroot/beet soup. Veal chop. Broccoli. Mango *or* peaches.

Day 3

Breakfast Hot brown rice *or* rice porridge with currants. Soy milk sweetened with dried fig *or* honey.

Lunch Split pea and ham soup. Cucumber boats with raw peanut butter and ground sunflower seeds. Grapes.

Dinner Turkey, prawns/shrimps *or* scallops. Sweet potato. Green beans. Blended banana/tofu dessert *or* slice of paw paw/papaya.

Drinks and snacks Diluted fresh grape juice. Rice cakes with mashed banana. Carrot sticks.

Day 4

Breakfast Thickened apples (tapioca flour). Almond milk. Eggless potato pancake (if desired).

Lunch Mashed potato with sardines. Mint and cabbage salad.

Dinner Lamb brains *or* lamb chop. Brussels sprouts, cauliflower *or* swede/rutabaga. Spinach. Strawberries *or* avocado slices.

Drinks and snacks Diluted fresh apple, apricot *or* orange juice or coconut milk which may be mixed with fruit juice. Orange segments. See 'Dairy Alternatives' section for other drink ideas based on nuts, seeds, and soy milk.

Foods found in Diet Plan No. 10, 'School Lunch Ideas', are often suitable for toddlers.

FOUR DAY ROTATION DIET PLAN No. 10
SCHOOL LUNCH IDEAS

Day 1

Example 1 Corn on the cob *or* crab and rice salad. Walnuts. Honeydew melon.

Example 2   100% rye bread sandwich with chopped chicken salad (bind with tahini). Watermelon wedges.

Example 3   Lentil soup *and/or* cold chicken sausages (wheat free). Home made popcorn. Kiwi fruit/gooseberries.

Example 4   Rice cakes with hummus spread. Hard-boiled egg. Celery sticks. Pineapple.

Day 2

Example 1   Rollmop (pickled herring). Raw salad with capsicum/red or green pepper slices. Handful cashews. Plums or prunes.

Example 2   Tomatoes stuffed with cooked flaked fish, capsicum/red or green pepper, shallots and salad dressing with a handful of pine nuts. Mandarin *or* berries.

Example 3   Cold veal chop *or* sausages (wheat free). Raw salad. Dates and cashews. Fresh *or* dried mango.

Example 4   Beef stock soup *or* bolognaise in a vacuum flask. Pistachio *or* pine nuts. Peach *or* pear.

Day 3

Example 1   Prawn/shrimp rice salad. Fresh *or* dried figs. Fresh *or* dried banana.

Example 2   Half rockmelon/cantaloupe. Rice cakes with nut butter and grated carrot. Roasted sunflower seeds.

Example 3   Cold fried rice with bacon, peas, toasted sunflower seeds, carrots, mushrooms. Grapes.

Example 4   Kidney bean soup. Paw paw/papaya fruit salad with pecan nuts.

Day 4

Example 1   Potato salad with sardines *or* lamb. Apple *or* cherries.

Example 2   Cold lamb chops with avocado *or* asparagus salad. Almonds *or* strawberries.

Example 3   Lamb shanks/shoulder-shank end soup with buckwheat noodles. Minted cauliflower salad. Orange.

Example 4   Fish rissoles. Spinach salad. Brazil nuts. Fresh *or* dried apricots.

To compile salads, consult dietary selection chart for vegetables of the day. Virtually any vegetable can be chopped or grated into a salad eg. pumpkin, turnip, parsnip, broccoli etc.

FOUR DAY ROTATION DIET PLAN No.11 INFANTS 6-12 MONTHS

Day 1
Breakfast   Pears, mashed *or* stewed. Bream/sea bass/porgy fillets soup (otional).

Lunch   Homemade beef stock soup/stew with pumpkin and parsley.

Dinner   Steamed bream/sea bass/porgy fillets. Zucchini/courgettes. Jelly/gelatin made from agar and diluted pineapple juice.

Day 2
Breakfast   Sago and prune juice (from prunes soaked 2 days in the refrigerator).

Lunch   Fresh mango pulp *or* jelly. Chicken liver (from free range chickens only) *or* steamed chicken purée.

Dinner   Thick chicken soup with tomato and celery. Jelly/gelatin made from agar and diluted prune juice.

Day 3
Breakfast   Rice cereal. Mashed banana.

Lunch   Tofu. Beans. Sweet potato.

Dinner   Turkey breast *or* fish with carrots. Paw paw/papaya. Jelly/gelatin made from agar and diluted grape juice.

Day 4
Breakfast   Avocado *or* stewed apple thickened with tapioca flour.

Lunch   Lamb's brains *or* spinach soup. (Blend avocado, spinach, parsley with meat stock).

Dinner   Lamb chop. Mashed potato and avocado. Jelly/gelatin made from gelatin and diluted orange or apple juice.

Baby food does not always have to be cooked. The juice of fruit and vegetables listed may be obtained with a juicer or by grating the food and pressing out the juice through gauze. Dilute before giving to the baby.

Breast-feeding mothers should also follow a rotation diet.

FOUR DAY ROTATION DIETARY SELECTION
VEGETARIAN

Day 1

Primary protein Eggs.

Seeds and nuts Macadamia, almonds.

Beans Nil.

Grains Rice, sago.

Fruits Pineapple, coconut, dates, apricots, cherries, peaches, plums, strawberries, persimmon, honeydew melon, watermelon.

Vegetables Onion, shallots, broccoli, Brussels sprouts, horseradish, watercress, turnip, potato, cucumber.

Cooking suggestions Coconut oil, kudzu (thickener), almond oil, rice vinegar, rice syrup.

Day 2

Primary protein Fish roe (eggs).

Seeds and nuts Peanuts, sesame seeds, pine nuts.

Beans Lima beans, chick peas/garbanzos.

Grains Corn (cornmeal, cornstarch), tapioca.

Fruits Fig, kiwifruit/gooseberries, mulberry, grapefruit, lemon, lychee, grape, raisin.

Vegetables Beetroot/beet, spinach, mushrooms, alfalfa, fennel, parsnip, nasturtium, avocado, olives.

Cooking suggestions Corn oil, sesame oil, olive oil, tahini, corn syrup, wine vinegar.

Day 3

Primary protein Quail eggs.

Seeds and nuts Filbert, cashew, pistachio, hazelnut.

Beans Nil.

Grains Rice, buckwheat, arrowroot.

Fruits Rhubarb, apple, pear, quince, blackberry, raspberry, mango, rockmelon/cantaloupe.

Vegetables   Tomato, eggplant/aubergine, capsicum/red or green pepper, asparagus, leek, chives, garlic, capers, cauliflower, cabbage, mustard greens, radish, pumpkin, zucchini/courgettes.

Cooking suggestions   Maple syrup, apple cider vinegar.

Day 4

Primary protein   Nil.

Seeds and nuts   Walnut, pecan, sunflower seed, linseed.

Beans   Kidney beans, lentils, soybeans (tofu, soy flour, soy grits, soy milk).

Grains   Rye, millet, oats, barley.

Fruits   Custard apple, paw paw/papaya, lime, orange, tangerine, guava, blueberry, banana.

Vegetables   Sweet potato, bamboo shoots, mung beans, carrot, celery, parsley, mint, lettuce/Webb's wonder/iceberg.

Cooking suggestions   Sugar, agar, carob, safflower oil, soy oil.

FOUR DAY ROTATION DIET PLAN No. 12
VEGETARIAN

Day 1

Breakfast   Prunes and sago with almond milk. Potato pancakes.

Lunch   Fruit salad with brown rice and coconut cream, topped with macadamia nuts.

Dinner   Omelette with shallots. Jacket baked potato. Broccoli. Watercress salad.

Day 2

Breakfast   Half grapefruit. Corn on the cob.

Lunch   Hummus with corn chips, fennel sticks and parsnip wedges. Kiwi fruit/gooseberries.

Dinner   Borscht soup. Avocado with olives and fish roe. Baby lima delight (topped with 'crust' of toasted sesame seeds).

Day 3

Breakfast   Hot brown rice with cashew milk and stewed pears. Buckwheat pancakes (eggless).

Lunch   Pumpkin soup. Rice crakers with cashew paste, asparagus and tomato. Rockmelon/cantaloupe balls.

Dinner   Ratatouille with 100% buckwheat noodles. Green salad. Apple and rhubarb crumble with cashew cream.

Day 4

Breakfast   Ground roasted barley cereal with banana/soy milk. Half paw paw/papaya.

Lunch   Kidney bean soup. Tofu 'cutlets'. Parsley-mint salad.

Dinner   Lentil casserole. Millet. Sweet potato. Lettuce salad. Tofu blueberry whip.

RICE DIET PLAN No. 13

• Incorporates rice as a staple food every day

Day 1

Breakfast   Slice of paw paw/papaya. Cooked brown rice with stewed apple and currants. Soy *or* fig milk.

Lunch   Rice salad with salmon or tuna, bean sprouts, carrot, asparagus *or* lentil casserole with rice (parsnips, carrot, celery, onion).

Dinner   Split pea soup. Asian style fish (sesame oil, tamari, garlic, shallots, carrot, celery, peas, beans). Boiled rice. Fresh *or* baked pear with fig cream.

Snacks   Rice cakes with peanut butter, grapes, raisins, walnuts, peanuts.

Cooking suggestions   Soy oil, sesame oil, fish oils.

Day 2

Breakfast   Slice of any melon. Cooked brown rice with dates and sunflower seed milk (blend dates and sunflower seeds with water). Goat's yogurt (if allowed).

Lunch   Borscht soup (beets, pumpkin, brown rice, meat if desired). *or* stuffed squash/marrow/winter squash (rice, minced meat, pine nuts).

Dinner   Half an avocado. Small portion of red meat with rice, pumpkin, zucchini/courgettes. Kiwi fruit/gooseberries.

Snacks Rice cakes with avocado butter, pumpkin seeds, melon slices, olives.

Cooking suggestions Olive oil.

Day 3

Breakfast Cooked brown rice with fresh *or* stewed apricots, peaches *or* stewed prunes. Almond milk.

Lunch Corn on the cob. Fruity rice salad (coconut, apricots, peaches, pineapple, almonds, Brazil nuts).

Dinner Stir-fried prawns/shrimps with Chinese cabbage, broccoli, cauliflower, water chestnuts. Boiled brown rice.

Snacks Rice cakes with almond butter, Brazil nuts, cherries, plums, dried apricots.

Cooking suggestions Corn oil, almond oil.

Day 4

Breakfast Cooked brown rice with sliced banana and raisins. Cashew milk.

Lunch Stuffed tomatoes (rice, sunflower seeds, pistachio nuts, capsicum/red or green pepper, lettuce cups/Webb's wonder/iceberg). Vegetable compote on brown rice (tomato, capsicum/red or green pepper, eggplant/aubergine, capers).

Dinner Artichoke hearts. Baked chicken *or* turkey breast with brown rice and salad (lettuce and orange with hard-boiled egg). Fresh slices of mango *or* orange.

Snacks Rice cakes with cashew butter *or* hazelnut butter. Buckwheat and hazelnut pancakes. Sunflower seeds. Oranges.

Cooking suggestions Safflower oil.

Further suggestions Use organically grown brown rice if possible. Substitute savory for sweet rice in the morning. Try a Japanese macrobiotic breakfast of miso soup and brown rice. Miso, a paste made from soybeans, is available at health food stores. Add a tablespoon to a pot of vegetable consommé before serving. Add mushrooms, shallots and sea vegetables. Make a point of chewing each mouthful very well to benefit fully from the rice diet.

SUBSTITUTES FOR COMMON FOODS

Dairy Products   page 97

Wheat Products   page 102

Eggs   Three eggs in a recipe can be replaced by:

1 tablespoon (20 ml/¾ fl oz) vinegar

1 tablespoon golden syrup/light corn syrup

1 tablespoon gelatin (dissolve in a little water and reduce recipe
liquid by this amount).

In biscuits/cookies, 1 egg can be replaced by 2 tablespoons (40 ml)
water, 1 tablespoon oil and 2 tablespoons baking powder.

In puddings/desserts, eggs can be replaced by 1 tablespoon gelatine
per 2 cups of liquid.

Oatmeal   Rice flakes, soya flakes, millet flakes.

Nuts   Seeds (sunflower, sesame, pine, pumpkin), sprouted seeds and
grains (see the range in a health food store).

Peanut butter   Cashew paste, almond paste, hazelnut paste. To
make tahini butter, mix equal portions of tahini (sesame paste) with
nut butter and a taste of honey. Also bean dips and purées.

Vegemite/marmite   Mix one third of miso paste with two thirds
tahini (sesame paste).

Soy sauce   Wheat-free tamari (natural soy sauce).

Sugar   Honey, pure maple syrup, rice syrup, date sugar, coconut,
blended dried fruit. In cooking, 1 cup of sugar equals approximately
two thirds a cup of honey. Less liquid is usually required when using
honey. Reduce baking temperature slightly and cook a little longer.
When using honey in large amounts, add ½ teaspoon bicarbonate
of soda/baking soda, per cup of honey.

Jelly(Jello)/Gelatin   Agar for preference, or gelatine and natural fruit
juices, fruits and nut milks.

Chocolate   Carob powder.

Soup Stock   Homemade from bones and vegetables, miso paste (a
substitute for beef stock), kelp liquid, protein powders.

Salad Dressings   See recipe section (Salads).

Tea and Coffee   Herbal teas, Japanese green tea, grain coffee.

DAIRY SUBSTITUTES

COCONUT MILK

1 teaspoon (5 ml) honey
1 cup water
⅓ cup dessicated coconut/shredded coconut
or *1 cup freshly ground coconut*

If using dessicated/shredded coconut, add boiling water to the coconut, let stand for half an hour, then squeeze out with a cheesecloth. Repeat this process for a weaker milk. If frozen, the milk will keep for months, otherwise it will keep only a few days. Use on cereals or in cooking.

AVOCADO CREAM

1 tablespoon (20 ml/¾ fl oz) honey
½-1 avocado
1 banana
Blend all ingredients. Serve with fruit salad.

TAHINI AND HONEY CREAM

Blend equal amounts of honey and tahini paste. Gradually add water until desired consistency is achieved, from thick to runny. Vanilla may be added. Serve with fruit salad or grains.

TOFU CREAM

Blend a packet of tofu with the fruit of your choice and a little honey.

ALMOND MILK OR CREAM

2 teaspoons (10 ml) honey (or to taste)
1 cup raw almonds
2½ cups water (less for cream)
Roughly chop almonds and blend dry. Gradually add water and honey to form the desired consistency.
Variations:
Add 1 green apple (omit honey)
Add carrot juice (2-4 carrots)
Add dessicated/shredded coconut and a small amount of lemon juice.
Add carob (1 tablespoon per cup)
Chop dates into almond cream, garnish with nuts or coconut.
Add sunflower seeds for a higher protein value.

ALMOND BUTTER

Prepare recipe (see page 99) for cashew butter. Similar butters can
be made from hazelnuts, Brazil nuts, etc.

SOY MILK

May be purchased in liquid or dry form from health food and oriental
shops, or prepared from soy beans.

CASHEW BUTTER

Blend one cup of ground cashews powdery fine. Gradually add 1
tablespoon (20 ml/¾ fl oz) of cold pressed oil of your choice to create
a smooth paste. Add a little salt to taste. Store in an airtight bottle
in the refrigerator.

CASHEW ICECREAM

3 cups nut cream
honey to taste
¼ cup cold pressed vegetable oil
3 cups fruit (eg strawberries, oranges, bananas, mangoes, dates)
2 tablespoons (40 g/1¼ oz) agar (optional)
Blend nut cream, honey and oil together. Blend or stir in fruit. Add
agar, dissolved in a little water over heat, if desired. Freeze the
mixture. When nearly frozen, beat again and refreeze.

CASHEW MILK

1 cup raw cashews
2½ cups water (or to taste)
1 teaspoon (5 ml) honey (or to taste)
vanilla (optional)

Blend dry cashews to form a meal. Gradually add water and honey to form first a thick paste and then a milky consistency.

Variations:

Add 1 banana

Add dates

Add both banana and dates

Add 1 tablespoon carob (20 g/¾ oz) per cup

Add soaked dried figs or fig juice

Add an apple

Add mangoes in season

CASHEW CREAM

Make as for cashew milk but do not add the same amount of water. Similar variations may be tried as above.

MOCK CREAMS AND ICINGS

125 g/4 oz copha

1 cup 155 g/5 oz icing sugar

1 teaspoon (5 ml) vanilla

1 tablespoon (20 ml/¾ fl oz) hot water

Have copha at room temperature. Chop roughly, then place in small warmed bowl with icing sugar. Beat until light and fluffy. Beat in vanilla and water. Spread or pipe onto cooked cake.

125 g/4 oz dairy free margarine

4 tablespoons (80 ml/2½ fl oz) honey

1 tablespoon (20 ml/¾ fl oz) water

vanilla or carob

Beat margarine until light and add honey one tablespoon at a time. Add water. Beat until creamy.

Variations:

1-2 tablespoons soymilk may be added to create a thicker icing.

Add chopped pineapple pieces and crushed nuts or other fruits or nuts for special tastes.

SOY MAYONNAISE

1 cup tofu (approximately 200 g/6½ oz)
1 small onion
1 clove garlic
1 teaspoon honey
½ teaspoon salt
3 tablespoons (60 ml/2 fl oz) lemon juice (or less)
¼ cup oil, cold
paprika to taste

Blend all ingredients except oil and lemon juice. Gradually add a trickle of oil while blending. Add lemon juice until the desired consistency has been reached.

TOFU CHEESECAKE

3 cups tofu (600 g/19 oz)
1 tablespoon tahini (20 g/¾ oz)
¾ cup (8 oz) raw honey
1 tablespoon (20 g/¾ oz) carob powder
1 teaspoon vanilla
½ teaspoon cinnamon
¼ teaspoon cloves

Combine ingredients well by hand. Pour into crust (see baking section) or individual dessert dishes. Chill before serving.

ICE CREAM

See dessert recipe section (page 172) for gelato, nutmilk, icecreams, sorbets.

SOY MILK CUSTARD

Substitute lactose free soy milk for cow's milk in favourite custard recipes. Thicken with extra soy milk powder.

DAIRY SUBSTITUTES IN COOKING

In baked products try using apple or orange juice instead of dairy products. For sauces calling for milk, or cream, try water, stock, or fruit juices.

WHEAT SUBSTITUTES

Flour   Cornstarch/cornflour, barley and rye flours, potato flour, soya flour and soya meal, lentil and bean flours, arrowroot, and tapioca flour.

For one cup of wheat flour try substituting:
- ½ cup (60 g/2 oz) soya flour and ½ cup cornflour/cornstarch
- ½ cup soya flour and ½ cup arrowroot
- ¾ cup (90 g/3 oz) rice flour
- ¾ cup potato flour
- ½ cup (60 g/2 oz) rice flour and ¼ cup (30 g/1 oz) potato flour

Bread and Sandwiches   Rice Bread, Sweet Pumpkin Bread, Sweet Buckwheat Bread, Copha Bread, Potato Bread, Quick Soya Bread. You may also use commercially available 100% rye bread, rye crackers and rice cakes.

Pasta   100% buckwheat noodles, rice vermicelli, bean threads, tacos.

Breadcrumbs   Crushed cereals or potato chips, millet meal, rice bran, ground nuts or seeds.

Baking Powder   Combine 45 g/1½ oz allowable flour, 30 g/1 oz cream of tartar, 52 g/1¾ oz bicarbonate of soda/baking soda, 30 g/1 oz tartaric acid. Rub mixture through a sieve twice. Store in airtight jar.

Some commercially available baking powders are wheat free.

RECIPES (wheat and dairy product free)

BREAKFASTS

BROWN RICE AGAIN

1 cup cooked brown rice, hot or cold
½ cup stewed sundried apricots or apple
almond or cashew milk

POTATO CAKE

oil
potato
onion (optional)

Heat about 1 tablespoon (20 ml/¾ fl oz) of cold-pressed oil in non-stick pan. Add grated potato and flatten into a round cake, similar in shape to an omelette. Cook one side till golden brown then turn carefully over and cook second side. Grated onion may be mixed with grated potato.

GENERAL WAFFLE RECIPE

2 cups cornmeal (maize meal, polenta)
2 teaspoon baking powder (wheat free)
2-3 eggs
2 cups water

Beat the ingredients together to form a thin batter. Preheat the waffle iron and grease for each waffle. Spoon the batter onto the iron until it covers the surface. Close and cook for 2 minutes. Transfer to a warm oven shelf to dry, not onto a plate which will make it soggy. Stir the mixture well before spooning onto the waffle iron as cornmeal will sink to the bottom of the bowl.

Variations:

Substitute buckwheat flour or rice flour. Add coconut, ground nuts, marzipan meal, grated carrot, or vanilla. Sweet foods like honey or sugar make these waffles stick to the iron. These waffles replace toast and can also be used for sandwiches.

RICE WAFFLES

1 cup brown rice flour
½ cup rice bran
1½ cups nut milk
½ teaspoon (2.5 ml) honey

1 tablespoon (20 ml/¾ fl oz) oil
2 eggs

Beat the ingredients together to form a thin batter. Preheat waffle iron and grease for each waffle. Spoon the batter onto the iron until it covers the surface. Close and cook for 2 minutes. Transfer to warm oven shelf to dry, not onto a plate which will make it soggy. Stir mixture well before spooning onto waffle iron as the flour sinks to the bottom of the bowl.

GENERAL PANCAKE RECIPE

2 cups flour of your choice
  - *buckwheat (light, dark)*
  - *corn (maizemeal, polenta)*
  - *rice flour (white or brown) in combination with rice bran OR grated potato, OR grated carrot with parsley.*
2 beaten eggs
2 tablespoons (30 g/1 oz) ground nuts
1½ cups water
2 teaspoons baking powder
1 tablespoon oil
cinnamon (optional)

Mix flour of your choice and water, baking powder, oil, and eggs to form a thin batter. Cook a spoonful at a time on a greased frypan or griddle, turning to cook both sides.

Variation:

Add more water to form a thinner batter. Serve a plain pancake with stewed fruit, fried or fresh banana, tahini/fruit sauces or nut cream.

BLENDER POTATO PANCAKE

¼ cup water
2 eggs
3 cups diced raw potato
1 small onion, chopped or a tablespoon dried onion flakes

3 tablespoons (30 g/1 oz) buckwheat flour or other—cornmeal,
rice etc.

pinch salt (optional)

½ teaspoon baking powder.

Put all the ingredients in order of listing into a blender. Cover and blend on chopping speed for 10 seconds or just until all potatoes go through the blender blades. Do not overblend or potatoes will be liquefied. Pour a small amount onto a greased griddle. These may also be cooked in a waffle iron.

EGGLESS PANCAKE

To cook a pancake mixture without eggs, use a small base frying pan, grease well, and pour mixture into the pan to cover bottom 1/10" (2.5 mm). Cover the pan with a lid, place on a low heat and cook, then loosen with a knife and tip out onto a plate.

APPLE SUNRISE

1 grated apple

1 tablespoon (7 g/¼ oz) crushed nuts

1 teaspoon sunflower seeds

a few dates

juice of 1 fresh orange (or other freshly prepared juice)

1 tablespoon (20 ml/¾ fl oz) almond or cashew cream

1 teaspoon dessicated/shredded coconut

Place grated apple in a dish and top with other ingredients. Use fresh pear, banana, peaches, etc. instead of apple.

CORN ON THE COB

1 piece fresh corn, boiled

1 teaspoon cold pressed safflower or sunflower oil, or equivalent

Spread over the corn with vegetable salt to taste.

SMOKED KIPPERS

1 smoked kipper per person
Heat kippers thoroughly in 2½ cm water. Bring to the boil in frying pan (this removes excess salt in kippers).

PAW PAW/PAPAYA

One generous slice of fresh paw paw/papaya.
Squeeze with lime or lemon juice.

FRUIT SALAD TAHINI

combination of fresh fruit in season: apple, pineapple, paw paw, passionfruit, strawberries, mango, banana, cherries, kiwi fruit/ gooseberries, watermelon, rockmelon/cantaloupe, etc.
tahini
honey
water
To make a sauce blend equal parts of tahini and honey. Stir, gradually adding drops of water to achieve desired consistency. This can be done in a food processor.
Pour sauce over the fruit salad.

LAMB CHOP

One grilled lamb chop with pieces of grilled pineapple or tomato.

BUCKWHEAT PANCAKES

1½ cups buckwheat
¾ cup arrowroot
1½ cups water

Grind buckwheat together to make a fine flour. Mix together with arrowroot. Stir in water. Add a little more water (about ⅛ cup), enough to make a good pouring consistency. Pour a small amount of the mixture into a greased pan. Cook well on both sides. Serve with stewed apple, or a variety of fruit sauces.

Variation:

Add mashed bananas or ground hazelnuts to the mixture.

HAZELNUT-BUCKWHEAT PANCAKE

1 cup buckwheat flour
2 tablespoons (15 g/½ oz) ground hazelnuts
¼ teaspoon salt
¼ teaspoon cinnamon
1 egg
3 cups water

Stir a well beaten egg into the sifted dry ingredients. Slowly add water to form a smooth batter. Heat a heavy oiled frypan to medium temperature and just cover the surface with batter. Fry until brown then turn carefully and fry the other side.

Variations:

Add ½ cup more water to form thinner crepes. Serve with stewed apple, fried bananas, tahini or nut creams as described in the dairy substitutes section.

COOKED CEREAL

Buckwheat and sago (soak overnight).

Cornmeal, maize meal, polenta, corn grits, rice. Cook these with water to the desired consistency, using 1 cup of cereal to 2-3 cups water.

Consider rotating millet, ground millet and linseed, roasted ground barley (toast under griller/broiler and grind finely), rolled oats and scotch oats.

Top with nut milk sweetened with honey, or nutmilk blended with banana, apple, pears, pineapple, dates, raisins, sultanas/seedless raisins, prunes. Also add crushed nuts, fresh fruit (grated, sliced), stewed fruit, fruit juice, soaked dried fruits (prunes, apricots, etc.)

CHOPPED POPCORN

Substitute this for dry cereal. Follow directions on packet for popping corn. Vary by popping with honey or mixing with nuts.

THICKENED APPLES

4 apples, peeled and chopped, stewed with ½ cup water
mix 1 oz/30 g maize or cornmeal with water and add to the hot
  apples
cook to thicken the mixture
add ½ teaspoon mixed spice

Substitute buckwheat flour, cornflour (cornstarch), tapioca flour, barley flour. Substitute pears, fresh apricots, fresh peaches.

BUBBLE AND SQUEAK

Left over vegetables, chopped
2 cups fresh cabbage
parsley or sprouts
1 onion
eggs

Lightly fry onion and cabbage, add cooked vegetables and heat through. Stir in parsley or sprouts. Served with poached egg or beat egg(s) and add to the mixture. Stir. Add ground pepper. Use this recipe on your egg day to use up any leftover 'safe' foods.

SCRAMBLED EGGS

1 small onion (finely sliced)
2 cups of mung bean sprouts, small handful parsley, chopped
2 eggs, lightly beaten

Lightly fry the onions, then add the bean sprouts or parsley and lastly the beaten eggs. May be eaten with papadams (Indian rice flour crackers).

CORN PONES FOR ANY MEAL, AM OR PM

1 cup cornmeal (stone ground, not polenta)
¼ cup raw nut butter
2 tablespoons (15 g/½ oz) sesame seed
2 tablespoons sprouts, grated carrot or mixture of other grated
  vegetables to taste, including onions.
pinch sea salt
1 tablespoon (15 ml/½ fl oz) corn oil

Mix in about ½ cup of hot water. Make flat pones 2.5 cm/1" thick and 7.5 cm/3" across. Cook on an oiled tray at 180°C/350°F/Gas 4 for ½ hour.

CORNMEAL BREAD OR PANCAKES

2 cups cornmeal
½ cup soyflour, or substitute
2 teaspoons baking powder
½ cup water
1 carrot
3 dates (or more to taste)
3 tablespoons (22 g/¾ oz) pumpkin seeds or sunflower seeds
2 tablespoons (15 g/½ oz) sesame seeds
½ cup oil
1-2 eggs
pinch salt

Combine cornmeal, soyaflour and baking powder in bowl. Place in the blender in order – water, carrot, seeds, oil, salt, eggs and blend well. Add to the dry ingredients. The batter should be stiff. Cook in greased nut roll tin at 150°C/300°F/Gas 2, for about 1 hour, or until skewer comes out clean.

Variations:
Use rye flour instead of cornmeal. Make batter thinner for pancake mix by using more eggs and eliminating the oil. Substitute nuts for seeds. Ground nuts may completely replace cornmeal in a pancake mix.

SUPER DRINK

Blend the following ingredients:
2 tablespoons (40 g/1¼ oz) soya milk powder
1 teaspoon lecithin
1 tablespoon (20 ml/¾ fl oz) honey
dash pure vanilla (optional)
1 egg (optional)
1 piece fruit in season, pear, apple, etc.
2 cups cold water
1 tablespoon (7 g/¼ oz) sunflower seeds.
1 tablespoon tahini (optional or to taste)
ground nuts to taste
Vary ingredients according to rotation plan.

BREAKFAST MUESLI

It is better not to pre-mix the muesli. Prepare individual ingredients:
cereal: raw or toasted or cooked if required
seeds: sunflower, sesame, pumpkin
fruits: Fresh, canned or stewed
diluted juice or nut milk
nuts: raw, or toasted (chopped or ground if desired)

Choose an item from each group (depending on the day) and allow children to make up their own muesli. (Supervision may be needed depending on age, to ensure a balance of ingredients.) On cold days, cereal can be cooked and nuts, fruit, etc added before eating.

TSAMPA (GROUND ROASTED BARLEY)

Take a desired quantity of barley and spread it evenly over griller (broiler) tray. Toast under medium heat, turning every minute or two, being careful not to burn the barley. Barley should be a rich brown colour. When cool, grind the roasted barley finely and then cook as porridge. Large quantities may be roasted, but more goodness is retained if the barley is ground just before cooking.

CRUNCHY RICE GRANOLA

6 cups rice flakes
1¼ cups soya flour
½-1 cup chopped nuts
¼ cup sunflower seeds
¾ cup dates
1½ cups water
⅓ cup oil
1 teaspoon salt
1 tablespoon (20 ml/¾ fl oz) honey
Blend dates, honey, oil and water in a food processor. Combine remaining ingredients. Add date mixture to dry ingredients. Mix well with fingers and crumble onto greased biscuit/cookie tray. Do not crumble too closely. Bake at 180°C/350°F for ten minutes and then reduce heat to 130°C/270°F/Gas 1 and bake a further 40 minutes or until dry.

SOUPS

CHICKEN SOUP

1 chicken carcass
2 tablespoons (15 g/½ oz) rice
1 chopped onion
2 stalks celery
3 cups water
½ cup apple juice
1 tablespoon (20 ml/¾ fl oz) cider vinegar
salt and pepper
parsley.

Break up carcass and simmer for about two hours with rice, onion, celery and vinegar. Remove bones and blend other ingredients. Add apple juice and simmer a further 5 minutes. Season. Serve with chopped parsley.

MUSHROOM AND BARLEY SOUP

1 cup barley
4 pints vegetable or chicken broth
1 onion
2 sprigs parsley
2 stalks celery
Cook the above ingredients for 1½ hours. Then add:
1-2 chopped carrots
500 g (1 lb) mushrooms
tamari soy sauce
Cook for another 20 minutes.
Variation:
Stir in miso paste before serving.

MISO SOUP

May be used like beef extract to flavour soups or as a soup on its own with small pieces of shallot to garnish. Made from soy beans, miso is excellent for forming beneficial intestinal bacteria.

RICE SOUP

1 clove garlic crushed
1 tablespoon (20 ml/¾ fl oz) oil
125 g/4 oz cooked rice
4 zucchini/courgettes
1-2 chopped tomatoes
1 litre/24 fl oz stock (chicken, fish, vegetable)
Sauté garlic in margarine or oil. Add cooked rice and zucchini. Sauté until golden. Add chopped tomatoes and stir. Add stock, bring to the boil and allow to simmer for 20 minutes. Season to taste.

BORSCHT

2-3 beets
1 onion
vegetables of choice (eg carrot, potatoes, cabbage, tomato.)
  equivalent to beets
½ teaspoon dill seeds, ground (or fresh dill if available)
1 litre/24 fl oz chicken or vegetable stock, or water
1 tablespoon (10 g/⅓ oz) soy flour (optional)
lemon juice, or goat's yogurt

Sauté vegetables in ½ tablespoon oil for about 15 minutes. Add broth and simmer until tender. Add remaining ingredients and cook a further 10 minutes. Blend and serve with lemon juice or goat's yogurt, if allowed. (For a chunkier soup, grate or cube the vegetables and do not blend.)

SPLIT PEA

1 cup (185 g/6 oz) split peas
2 cups water
1 ham bone
vegetable salt
1 celery stick
small piece turnip (optional)
1 small onion
1 bay leaf
other herbs to taste

Simmer all ingredients for 1½-2 hours. Remove the ham bone. Blend in other ingredients. Cut meat off the bone and add to the soup.

Variations:

Add ½ cup chopped carrot, or ½ cup chopped parsley, or sea vegetables, eg kombu or wakame. Omit ham bone, and add 1 extra onion.

LENTIL SOUP

2 cups (370 g/12 oz) lentils
1 onion
1 tomato
2-3 carrots
3 stalks celery
salt or tamari soy sauce
Cover with water and boil until the lentils are tender. Blend.
Variations:
Using red lentils reduces cooking time to about 15 minutes. Add vegetables — steam potato chunks and large slices of cabbage for 10-15 minutes. Place in a bowl and pour the soup over. Add chicken pieces and pour soup over. Add bacon bones to soup mixture.

POTASSIUM BROTH

Celery, celery leaves, carrots, spinach, parsley, chives, fennel, leeks, turnip tops, carrot tops. Finely chopped or grated vegetables are most suitable.
Cook slowly for one hour in water to cover.

AVOCADO SOUP

Blend 2 avocados, 2 pints (1.25 litres) vegetable stock and 2 cups
goat's yogurt (or nut milk plus a little lemon juice).
Can be served hot or cold.

SCOTCH BROTH

1 kg/2 lbs stewing meat of your choice
2½ litres (4¼ pints) water
¼ cup pearl barley (or unpearled) soaked
¼ cup (45 g/1½ oz) soaked dried peas of your choice

3 onions or mixture of onions and leeks
1-2 carrots
1-2 turnips
½ small cabbage
parsley
salt
pinch nutmeg

Cover meat, barley and peas with cold water and bring to the boil. Add diced vegetables and simmer slowly for at least 2 hours. Add cabbage and seasonings and cook uncovered for 20 minutes. Vary meat and vegetables according to your rotation plan and seasonal availability.

MINESTRONE

onions
carrots
celery sticks
potatoes
zucchini/courgettes
green beans
cabbage
oil and margarine for sauté
5 cups of beef stock, or enough water to cover well
4 large ripe tomatoes or canned tomatoes
1 cup (185 g/6 oz) cannellini or borlotti beans (presoaked overnight)

Finely dice all vegetables and shred the cabbage. Heat the oil and margarine in a large pan, add onions, then potatoes, celery, zucchini, beans and cabbage. Cook each vegetable for about 3 minutes before adding the next. Add water, beef stock, beans and mashed tomatoes. Bring to the boil, and simmer (covered), until the soup is thick and the beans are well cooked (about 2 hours). Season with salt and pepper.

Traditionally, grated parmesan cheese is served with the soup.

ALMOND SOUP

5 cups (1.25 litres) strong chicken stock
2 onions chopped
2-3 large sliced old potatoes
salt
pepper
4 teaspoons grated orange rind
1 cup ground blanched almonds (not too powdered)
300 mls/10 fl oz nut cream
1 cup chicken (cooked)
1 diced avocado (optional)

Sauté onions and add to the chicken stock. Add potatoes and simmer until tender. Cool. Put into a blender and blend until smooth. Add orange rind, ground almonds, cream, chicken and avocado. Serve sprinkled with orange zest and parsley.

KIDNEY BEAN SOUP

300 g/10 oz beans
1 litre/1¾ pints water
1 stalk celery
1 large onion
½ green pepper/capsicum
black pepper

Soak beans overnight in water. Bring rapidly to boil. Boil for 5 minutes and then simmer until tender with celery, onion, green pepper and pepper. Blend. Add herb salt to taste, 1 tablespoon (20 ml/¾ fl oz) lemon juice and a dash of sherry. Garnish with lemon slices.

Variation:

Use chick peas/garbanzos, lima beans, pinto beans, butter beans/dried lima beans. Vary vegetables to include garlic, large amounts of parsley, cabbage and other fresh herbs such as basil, thyme or summer savory.

SALADS

SALAD NICOISE

1 lettuce/Webb's wonder/iceberg
250 g/½ lb green beans (lightly cooked)
250 g/½ lb potatoes (boiled and thickly sliced)
finely chopped parsley
2 hard-boiled eggs (optional)
1 small can tuna
65 g/2 oz black olives
250 g/½ lb tomatoes

All ingredients should be prepared in bite-sized chunks. Flake the tuna. Serve layered on a bed of lettuce with potatoes and beans, followed by tuna and tomatoes, then a layer of eggs, olives and parsley. Pour on an oil and vinegar dressing. In a rotation diet any of these ingredients could be omitted and others substituted, such as, cooked cauliflower, broccoli, capsicum/red or green pepper, celery, anchovies, capers.

CHICK PEA SALAD

1 cup dried chick peas/garbanzos, cooked
4 shallots
small handful parsley, chopped
¼ cup oil
2 tablespoon lemon juice
½ teaspoon salt
⅛ teaspoon mustard

Chop shallots and parsley finely. Mix with cooked chick peas. Make dressing with other ingredients and toss through salad. Serve on lettuce leaves.

Variation:
Use tahini instead of oil dressing. Add grated carrot or grated radish.

PARSLEY SALAD (TABOULI)

2 cups finely cut parsley
½ cup fresh mint
¼ cup (30 g/1 oz) sesame seeds
¼ cup sunflower seeds, toasted
1 onion, finely chopped or grated
2 tomatoes diced small (optional)
3 tablespoons olive oil
juice of 2 lemons

Mix oil and lemon juice. Toss the remaining 6 ingredients in the dressing.

Variations:
Instead of seeds use cooked buckwheat or millet. Use chives, shallots or garlic instead of onion.

GREEK SALAD

lettuce/Webb's wonder/iceberg
tomato wedges
thin onion rings
olives
olive oil
lemon juice or vinegar dressing
fetta cheese (optional)
Combine ingredients and top with a dressing of olive oil and lemon juice.

GREEK CABBAGE SALAD

700 g/1½ lb shredded cabbage
225 g/7 oz cooked haricot beans
4 tablespoons (80 ml/2½ fl oz) olive oil
3 tablespoons lemon juice
8 black olives
Combine oil and lemon juice to form a dressing. Toss remaining ingredients in dressing.

INDIVIDUAL AVOCADO AND MUSSEL SALADS

2 small avocados
18 mussels
2 tomatoes
8 black olives
4-5 sprigs parsley, finely cut
DRESSING
½ cup oil
2 tablespoon vinegar
1½ teaspoon ground cumin
½ teaspoon French mustard

salt, pepper
pinch sugar

Prepare mussels by washing shells. Steam in an open pan of water. Discard any which do not open. Place the mussels in bowl and pour over the prepared dressing, then leave until ready to serve. Cut avocados in half and peel gently. Slice the avocado halves lengthwise. Gently fan out slices on serving plates, allowing half an avocado per person. Brush avocado lightly with a little dressing from the mussles. Cut the tomatoes in half, slice thickly, and combine with olives and parsley. Drain dressing from mussels onto tomatoes, and mix lightly. Arrange 3 mussels on each serving plate and place a little of the tomato salad on each.

CALAMARI SALAD

400 g/13 oz cleaned calamari pieces
⅓ cup (85 ml/2½ fl oz) lemon juice
½ cup oil
1 small lettuce/Webb's wonder/iceberg
6 shallots
1 clove garlic
1 tablespoon salad dressing extra
salt, pepper

Cut the calamari into rings about 5 mm/¼" thick. Drop it into boiling water, reduce the heat and simmer 10-15 minutes, or until the squid is tender (depends on the size of the squid). Drain. Combine lemon juice and oil, add squid, mix well. Cover and refrigerate overnight. Next day drain the squid, and reserve the marinade. Place finely shredded lettuce, chopped shallots and squid in a large bowl. Combine reserved marinade with crushed garlic and salad dressing, salt, pepper and mix well. Pour over salad, toss well.

Variation:
Any herbs or green vegetables in the rotation plan.

AUTUMN SALAD

2 avocados
4 mandarins
4-5 sprigs chopped parsley, finely cut
½ cup salad dressing
½ lettuce/Webb's wonder/iceberg

Peel avocados, cut into slices. Break mandarins into segments. Remove pips. Combine parsley and the salad dressing, salt and pepper to taste. Put lettuce into the salad bowl with avocado slices. Toss. Garnish with mandarin slices.

MARINATED MUSHROOMS

250 g/½ lb small mushrooms
3 tablespoons lemon juice
½ cup oil (mixture of olive and other)
4-5 sprigs parsley, finely cut
¼ teaspoon salt
¼ teaspoon tarragon
Pepper

Slice mushrooms thinly. Prepare the dressing from the left over ingredients. Add mushrooms. Mix well. Cover and marinate mixture for 4 hours or overnight. This mixture is good when tossed through a green salad, with enough juice to coat the lettuce.

WALDORF SALAD

1 red apple
1 green apple
½ cup walnut pieces
1 cup finely chopped celery
juice of 1 lemon
¼ cup (60 ml/2 fl oz) soy mayonnaise
crisp lettuce leaves

Chop unpeeled apples into cubes and dip in the lemon juice. Combine all ingredients except the lettuce. Serve in lettuce cups *or* on a bed of fresh lettuce leaves.

ORIENTAL BEAN SALAD

½ cup cooked kidney beans
½ cup cooked soybeans
½ cup cooked green beans
½ cup mung bean sprouts
4 chopped shallots
1 grated carrot
⅓ cup peanut oil
2 tablespoons wine vinegar
ginger to taste
garlic to taste

Prepare dressing from peanut oil, wine vinegar, ginger and garlic. Combine other ingredients and pour over dressing. Refrigerate before use. Quantities need only be approximate.

SALAD COMBINATIONS

1 Lettuce, grated carrot, diced cucumber, diced apple, watercress, lemon juice.

2 Radish slices, chopped mint, lemon and oil dressing.

3 Bean sprouts, cooked soya beans, diced apples, mandarin segments, nuts, chives with tofu and lemon dressing.

4 Cooked beans, bean sprouts, green beans (cooked or raw), grated carrot, chopped capsicum/red or green pepper, celery, shallots in lemon/oil/honey dressing.

5 Watercress, sliced mushrooms, sliced carrot, chopped pineapple, pumpkin seeds, nuts, raisins, in spicy dressing (add ginger or cayenne to standard dressing.)

6 Lettuce, sliced avocado, sliced pear, raisins in dressing of oil, cider vinegar and salt.

7 Cooked lentils, shallots, parsley, white radish.

8 Cooked chick peas/garbanzos, diced capsicum/red or green pepper, shallots or chopped onion, grated carrot with dressing of tamari soy sauce/tahini/lemon juice, stirred slowly to a creamy consistency.

9 Shredded lettuce or cabbage, topped with grated carrot, grated beets, alfalfa sprouts, grated radish and cooked hijiki (seaweed), topped with tahini dressing and sunflower seeds.

10 Grated carrot, raw cabbage, grated parsnip, grated radish, grated onion, dressing, garnish of sprouts.

11 Chopped lettuce, grated cauliflower, radishes.

12 Fresh pineapple, red cabbage, parsley.

13 Thinly sliced onion, chicory/endive and spinach.

14 Mignonette lettuce/cabbage lettuce/boston/bibb lettuce, fennel slices, alfalfa sprouts, red pepper/capsicum slices.

15 Fill scooped out pineapple with mixture of pineapple, crabmeat, celery, walnuts, apple and a dash curry powder.

16 Coleslaw—homemade, with olive oil dressing.

17 Potato salad with soy mayonnaise or oil and vinegar dressing.

18 Mixture of mung bean sprouts, chopped celery, chopped shallots, garnished with hard-boiled eggs and fried onion rings, served with peanut butter/lemon juice/garlic/chilli dressing.

19 Cooked diced or raw grated beets, cooked diced pumpkin, grated carrot, grated turnip, grated parsnip, diced unpeeled apple, diced capsicum/red or green pepper, chopped onion, chives, grated cabbage, diced celery and diced fennel. Try these in winter salads.

20 For a pleasant change, spike your salad bowl with a tablespoon of minced fresh basil, watercress, chopped green pepper or fragrant mint leaves.

21 Add any of your favorite proteins to these salad ideas: ½ cup or more of tuna fish, salmon, sardines, chicken, turkey, hard boiled eggs, left over meats. Throw in a handful of sunflower seeds or toasted sesame seeds.

IDEAS FOR SALAD DRESSING

1   Blend oil and apple cider vinegar with a handful of parsley and chives from the garden. Salt and pepper to taste.

2   Asian dressing: 3 tablespoons (60 ml/2 fl oz) lemon juice, 3 tablespoons tamari, ½ cup (125 ml/4 fl oz) safflower oil, and a few drops of sesame oil.

3   3 tablespoons tahini, 1 cup water, 1 teaspoon kelp powder, juice of ½ lemon, small clove garlic. Blend the ingredients together.

4   Creamy bean dressing: 1 cup cooked beans (eg chick peas/garbanzos, pinto beans, etc), juice of 1 lemon, dash of tamari, 2 cloves garlic, 3 tablespoons safflower oil or tahini. This dressing is a high protein complement to a sprout salad.

5   Lemon juice, honey and mint.

6   Lime/lemon juice, garlic, oil, choice of hot spices eg. chili, ginger, cayenne.

7   Lemon juice, honey and a variety of nut butters.

8   Tofu dressing: 1 packet (200 g/6½ oz) tofu, 2 tablespoons (40 ml/1¼ fl oz) lemon juice, 3-4 tablespoons (60 ml/2 fl oz) unrefined oil *or* 2 tablespoons tahini, ½ teaspoon sea salt, 1 teaspoon wheat free tamari soy sauce, 1 small clove crushed garlic, or equivalent in minced onion, chives or shallots, 2 tablespoons minced parsley. Purée ingredients in blender except the parsley. Serve with sprinkled parsley. Serve over salads, as a dip with fresh vegetables, chips or cooked vegetables.

VEGETABLE DISHES

SWEET POTATO BAKE

2 large potatoes
2 carrots
6 prunes
1 cup water
1 apple, cubed

Cut sweet potato into cubes. Simmer with carrots and prunes for about 25 minutes. Add apple and cook a further 20 minutes. Bake uncovered for a further 20 minutes in a moderately hot 180°C/350°F/Gas 4 oven.

BEETROOT WITH LEMON SAUCE

½ kg/1 lb beetroot/beet, sliced
juice of 2 lemons
1 teaspoon grated lemon rind

1 teaspoon honey
salt (optional)
1 teaspoon arrowroot, dissolved in ½ cup beet liquid

Steam beetroot and reserve liquid. In another saucepan combine lemon juice, rind, honey, salt and arrowroot. Simmer slowly until thickened. Serve over beetroot.

Variation:

Slice and store remaining beetroot in a jar partially filled with cider vinegar for use in salads.

FRIED PARSNIPS

Clean parsnips and slice them lengthways in the smallest possible slices. Do not use core. Stand in hot water for 20 minutes (retain the water for other purposes), drain and wipe. Fry the parsnips quickly in vegetable oil. A couple of minutes should be adequate.

CHINESE VEGETABLES

1 onion
1 clove garlic
1 tablespoon oil
1 stick celery
750 g/1½ lb Chinese cabbage
½ cup water chestnuts
1 tablespoon tamari soy sauce

In a wok or heavy frypan sauté the chopped onion and garlic clove in vegetable oil. Add the finely sliced stick of celery, and the Chinese cabbage. Cook for two minutes. Add finely sliced water chestnuts, and tamari soy sauce. Put lid on wok and simmer for 5-10 minutes, stirring occasionally. Vegetables should remain crisp.

Variation:

Substitute other Chinese vegetables, or carrots, parsnips, turnips, etc.

BEANS IN SESAME SAUCE

250 g/½ lb green beans
1 cup water
½ cup (60 g/2 oz) sesame seeds
1 teaspoon honey
1 tablespoon tamari soy sauce

Halve and string the beans if desired. Place in boiling water with honey. Cover and steam for 5 minutes. Remove, drain and save the water. Fry the sesame seeds in a hot frypan for 1 minute, taking care not to burn them. When cool, grind to a moist powder. Pour sesame powder into bean stock. Cook for 2 minutes. Add beans and cook for 2 minutes more. Remove and serve with a sprinkling of sesame sauce over beans. Leftover beans make a delicious salad ingredient.

RATATOUILLE (VEGETABLE STEW)

2 eggplants/aubergines, sliced
2 zucchini/courgettes, sliced
3-4 tablespoons (60 ml/2 fl oz) olive oil
1 onion, sliced
2 cloves garlic
salt and pepper to taste
¼ kg/½ lb tomatoes, peeled and sliced
1-2 green peppers/capsicum, finely sliced

Eggplant can be salted to extract any bitterness (optional). Pat dry. Fry garlic, onion, eggplant and zucchini in hot oil until brown. Season. Add tomatoes and peppers, cover and cook for 1 hour (or until done). Serve hot or cold. Excellent with roast meat or barbecue.

Variations:
After the initial frying, cooking can be continued in a casserole, in a moderate oven 180°/350°F/Gas 4, until vegetables are soft but not mushy.

Serve with baked potato as this dish is predominantly 'potato family'.

Italian style: Omit zucchini and green pepper. Add 2-3 red

peppers/capsicum and 2 stalks of celery. Add final ingredients before slowly cooking; 1 tablespoon capers, several chopped black olives, 1 tablespoon sugar or 1 teaspoon (5 ml/½ fl oz) honey and 2 tablespoons vinegar.

SAUTÉED CAULIFLOWERETTES

Cook required amount of cauliflower until just barely tender. Break into small pieces and drain. Fry in non-dairy margarine or oil. Turn often. Serve sprinkled with ground roasted sesame seeds.

VEGETABLE KEBABS

500 g/1 lb small mushrooms
500 g/1 lb firm tomatoes or cherry tomatoes
1 red pepper/capsicum
1 green pepper/capsicum
small bunch spring onions, or onions, quartered
oil for basting
lemon juice
garlic salt

Wipe the mushrooms clean. Chop the peppers into chunks and blanch for a couple of minutes in boiling water. Drain. Thread all ingredients as desired on skewers. During cooking, baste kebabs with a mixture of oil, lemon juice and garlic salt, or use whole garlic if preferred. Kebabs may be slowly grilled or pan fried, basting frequently until cooked sufficiently.

Variations:

Use any vegetables in season. Hard vegetables such as carrots, cauliflower, etc may be blanched prior to preparation.

STAMP (POTATO AND VEGETABLE MASH)

1 kg/2 lb carrots
2 kg/4 lb potatoes
3 large onions
salt
water

Peel carrots, potatoes and onions. Cut into small pieces. Put in pot of water, add salt. Boil in water until tender. Drain most of the water off, leaving enough to make a nice moist mash. Mash.
Serve with plain fried pork ribs or a lamb goulash.

Variations:
Spinach/spring or collard greens can replace carrots and onions. Serve with savoury mince.
Sauerkraut toned down with cabbage can replace carrot and onions. Serve with pork.

RED PEPPERS WITH SPINACH

6 large red peppers/capsicum
250 g/8 oz spinach
2 tomatoes, coarsely chopped
2 anchovies
1 tablespoon oil
½ teaspoon black sugar

Remove seeds from peppers. Rub peppers with oil and grill/broil for about five minutes. Chop spinach finely and boil for a couple of minutes, drain and place in a pan with oil, tomatoes, sugar, and anchovies. Stir well during the cooking. When tomatoes are cooked, remove the mixture from the heat and stuff into peppers. Bake peppers in a slow oven 120°C/250°F/Gas ½ for 10 minutes.

STUFFED TOMATOES

4-6 firm ripe tomatoes
4 large stalks spinach
5 g/¼ oz pine nuts
1½ tablespoons oil
¾ cup cooked brown rice
1 clove garlic
¼ teaspoon basil or oregano
salt and pepper to taste

Cut tops off tomatoes, scoop out flesh and turn upside down to drain. Cook spinach, with stalks removed, for about 5 minutes until just tender. Roast pine nuts in half the oil until golden. Blend spinach and add the pine nuts. Blend again. Stir in seasonings, crushed garlic and remaining oil. Fold in rice. Spoon mixture into tomatoes. Bake in greased ovenproof dish at 180°C/350°F/Gas 4, about 15-20 minutes.

Variation:

Use this or a similar mixture to stuff vegetables, eg zucchini/courgette boats, partially cooked butternut pumpkin halves, etc.

RED CABBAGE

1 small red cabbage
1 tablespoon oil
250 ml/8 fl oz water
4 cloves
2 apples
1 tablespoon black sugar, or honey
2 tablespoons cider vinegar
salt to taste

Remove the core from the cabbage and shred very finely. Peel the core and slice apples. Combine oil, water, cabbage, cloves, salt and apples in a large saucepan. Cover and simmer for about 1 hour. Five minutes before serving time add the sugar and vinegar. Simmer.

POTATO SAMBAL

2 large potatoes, cooked and mashed
½ onion or shallot or chives
¼ red pepper/capsicum
1 tablespoon (7 g/¼ oz) dessicated/shredded coconut or equivalent
of coconut cream
3 tablespoons (60 ml/2 fl oz) soy milk
15 ml/⅔ fl oz oil

Combine soy milk, coconut, and oil in pan. Place onion, and pepper in mixture and simmer until soft. Add potatoes, and mix all the ingredients thoroughly. Serve as an accompaniment to curries or grills/broils.

STARTERS

Antipasta   *138*
Avocado fellini   *134*
Baba ghannouj   *138*
Broad bean purée   *139*
Cauliflower with mint   *138*
Corn on the cob   *135*
Dal   *137*
Devilled kidneys   *136*
Garlic prawns/shrimps   *135*
Gourmet's cocktail   *134*
Guacamole   *137*
Hummus   *135*
Lentil purée   *139*
Proscuitto melone   *140*
Rollmops   *140*
Russian bean dip   *137*
Squid marinated   *136*

AVOCADO FELLINI

Per person:
½ avocado pear
thin slice of pickled red pepper
3 black olives
Serve on a lettuce leaf with lemon juice or French dressing.

GOURMET'S COCKTAIL

Choose at least one seafood ingredient and add others to taste:
   ie prawns/shrimps, oysters, crab, scallops, tomato, celery slices,
   capsicum slices/red or green pepper, radishes, cucumber slices.

Serve on bed of chopped lettuce or alfalfa sprouts. Dress with lemon juice, soy mayonnaise, or French dressing.

HUMMUS

1 cup cooked chick peas/garbanzos
⅓ cup of tahini (sesame butter)
¼ cup lemon juice
1 large clove chopped garlic
½ teaspoon salt (optional)
Blend all together and serve as a dip, garnished with chopped parsley. Eat with a raw vegetable, such as celery, carrot, zucchini/courgettes; or corn chips or rice crackers.

CORN ON THE COB

Steam corn according to taste. Some people like it almost raw, others like it cooked for 10-15 minutes. May be served with cold-pressed safflower oil.

GARLIC PRAWNS

1 kg/2 lb green king prawns/shrimps
125 g/4 oz small mushrooms
1 red capsicum/red pepper
1 stick celery
4 cloves garlic
4 shallots
1 cup oil of your choice
250 g/8 oz margarine (or ½ cup olive oil)
salt
pepper
½ teaspoon/5 g chilli powder
Shell and clean prawns, leaving tails intact. Slice mushrooms, celery and capsicum thinly. Chop shallots. Place ¼ of the oil and margarine

(or olive oil) mixture into each of your individual oven proof dishes. Crush a clove of garlic into each dish, and add a pinch of chilli powder. Bake in hot oven 220°C/425°F/Gas 7, for 10 minutes. Divide remaining ingredients into 4 portions. Season with salt and pepper. Cook for further 10 minutes or until prawns are cooked.

SQUID MARINATED

500 g/1 lb squid (calamari)
⅓ cup lemon juice
⅓ cup oil
1 clove garlic
finely cut parsley to taste
Drop into rapidly boiling water and reduce heat. Simmer 10-15 minutes until tender. Drain. Combine juice and oil and add squid. Cool overnight. Next day add garlic and parsley. Let stand for 2 hours. Serve in marinade.

DEVILLED KIDNEYS

8 lamb kidneys (skinned, halved and core removed)
8 rashers bacon (trimmed and halved)
2 tomatoes (skinned and sieved)
1 teaspoon tomato paste
1 tablespoon (20 ml/¾ fl oz) tamari
small handful chopped parsley
Wrap kidneys in bacon and pack into a small ovenproof dish. Bake at 200°C/390°F/Gas 6, for approximately 30 minutes. Remove surface fat from juices and stir in tomato, tomato paste and tamari. Return to oven for 5 minutes. Serve sprinkled with parsley.
Variation:
Serve for breakfast

RUSSIAN BEAN DIP

6 cups cooked red kidney beans
2 chopped onions
2 tablespoon (40 ml/1¼ fl oz) oil
3 cloves garlic, crushed
dash of coriander
3 sprigs fresh dill, chopped
150-200 g/6-7 oz chopped walnuts

Blend beans. Sauté onions in oil, and add to the beans. Stir in remaining ingredients. Serve with raw vegetables and cornchips. This is also good as a sandwich spread.

GUACAMOLE

2 avocados, peeled and mashed
1 large peeled and chopped tomato
4 teaspoons lemon juice, or to taste
1 small finely chopped onion
1 crushed clove garlic

Mix all ingredients. Chili or tabasco can be added to give extra heat. Serve with raw vegetables, corn chips or rice crackers.

DAL

1½ cups (280 g/9 oz) lentils (washed and picked over)
4 cups water
2 tablespoons (40 ml/1¼ fl oz) oil
2 cloves garlic
salt
cayenne

Boil lentils in water until very soft, adding more water if necessary. Heat the oil in a skillet, adding garlic and lowering the heat. Remove the lentils from the water with a slotted spoon and place in oil. Stir and mash lentils in oil with enough cooking liquid to achieve the consistency of very thick soup. Add salt and cayenne. Cumin adds a more exotic taste.

BABA GHANNOUJ

1 large or 2 small eggplants/aubergines
3 cloves garlic
1 teaspoon salt
½ cup (125 g/4 oz) sesame paste (tahini)
¼ cup (60 ml/2 fl oz) strained lemon juice
olive oil
paprika

Bake eggplant. Cool and peel under running cold water, removing all skin. Blend. Gradually add crushed garlic, salt, tahini and lemon juice, to form thick mayonnaise consistency. Spread on a flat plate. Sprinkle oil over the surface and a little paprika around the edge.
Variation:
Add up to ½ cup chopped parsley to mixture.

ANTIPASTA

A cold Italian first course where a wide choice of ingredients can fit well into the frame of a rotation diet. Choose from olives, pickled vegetables, avocados, artichokes, capsicum/red or green pepper, tomatoes, anchovies, sardines, oysters, prawns/shrimps, capers, smoked salmon, salami, raw or pickled mushrooms, shallots, goats cheese. Arrange attractively on a bed of lettuce.

CAULIFLOWER WITH MINT

1 cauliflower
small handful chopped mint
1 clove garlic
½ cup olive oil

⅓ cup (85 ml/2½ fl oz) cider vinegar, or substitute
salt and pepper

When the cauliflower is cooked and cooled, toss it in a mixture of
mint, garlic and oil and refrigerate for approximately one hour.
Before serving, toss with vinegar and season with salt and pepper.

LENTIL PURÉE

225 g/7 oz cooked lentils, drained
4 tablespoons (80 ml/2¾ fl oz) lemon juice (or to taste)
2 cloves garlic, crushed
3 tablespoons (60 ml/2¼ fl oz) olive oil or peanut oil
fresh herbs as available

Drain the cooked lentils and blend with lemon juice and crushed
garlic. Add olive oil, stirring into a paste. Add fresh herbs. If the
mixture is too thin, add rice bran, mashed potato or arrowroot.

Variations:
Press into a paté shape and serve as a snack.
Deep fry in small round balls like falafel. Eat as an appetizer.
May be bound with an egg.
Add tahini and tamari instead of olive oil, or ground nuts, seeds
or grated carrot.

BROAD BEAN PURÉE

100 g/3¼ oz dried broad beans
5 bay leaves
1 lemon
2 cloves garlic, crushed
1 teaspoon aniseed, crushed
handful chopped parsley or mint
1 tablespoon (20 ml/¾ fl oz) olive oil
salt and pepper

Soak beans three times in boiling water. Allow to cool and discard water after each soaking. Add 500 ml/4 cups of cold water and simmer with bay leaves and lemon rind for 45 minutes. The beans should be mushy. Cool. Throw out bay leaves. Combine beans with garlic, lemon juice, aniseed and fresh herbs. Stir in olive oil and work the mixture into a paste.

ROLLMOPS (PICKLED HERRING)

Purchase rollmops at a delicatessen: 1 per person or ½ with potato side salad.

PROSCIUTTO MELONE

Purchase at a delicatessen: 2 slices prosciutto ham per person served with a generous slice of rockmelon/cantaloupe on a bed of lettuce.

RICE DISHES

BASIC FRIED RICE

2 cloves garlic
2 onions
4 shallots
1 small carrot
1 stick celery
1 cob of corn (optional)
handful of sunflower seeds
1 egg
3 cups precooked rice

Sauté onions and garlic for 5 minutes, then add finely diced carrot and celery. Cook for a further 2 minutes; then add seeds and shallots and sauté until brown. Add coarsely cut fried egg and rice and heat through. Before serving add tamari soy sauce to taste.

NASI GORENG

2 tablespoons (40 ml/1¼ fl oz) cooking oil
3 large onions
liberal sprinkle of chili powder (to taste)
¼ cup cooked prawns/shrimps, chopped
¼ cup diced cooked pork or chicken
¼ cup chopped mushrooms
4 cups cooked brown rice
tamari soya sauce to taste
3 beaten eggs (optional)
2 stalks celery, finely chopped

Slice the onions finely, reserve ¼ for adding later. Fry onions in the oil. When they are soft add the prawns, pork or chicken and mushrooms. Stir in the rice and add the chili powder and tamari sauce. If using eggs, add these and stir until they are cooked and the rice is dry. Add the remaining onion and celery.

SUMMER PAELLA

2 cups chicken stock
1 cooked chicken breast
250 g/½ lb brown rice
chicken stock and water
1 clove garlic
pinch saffron
salt and pepper
oil
3 shallots
½ red pepper/capsicum
½ green pepper/capsicum
60 g/2 oz cooked peas
250 g/½ lb king prawns/shrimps
good sprinkle chopped parsley
vinaigrette dressing

Gently fry garlic and brown rice in oil, for 3-4 minutes. Add chicken stock and water and cook the rice by absorption method, adding more water if necessary. Spread rice on a serving platter and allow to cool. Cover with peas, thinly sliced capsicum, chopped shallots, prawns and parsley. Sprinkle with enough dressing to moisten salad and toss gently.

PISTACHIO RICE

2 tablespoons (40 ml/1¼ fl oz) oil
2 cups cooked brown rice
1 onion
⅓ cup pistachio nuts or chopped almonds
½ teaspoon ground mace

Sauté onions in oil. Add nuts and sauté a further five minutes until lightly brown. Stir in rice and mace and heat through.

Variation:
Use sunflower seeds and garlic instead of pistachio nuts and onions. Omit mace, and add tamari soy sauce.

CURRIED LAMB AND RICE SALAD

1 chopped apple (sprinkled with lemon juice)
½ cup goat's yogurt (optional)
generous sprinkle curry powder (to taste)
¼ cup (60 ml/2 fl oz) soy mayonnaise
2-3 cups diced roast lamb
½ cup raisins
salt and pepper

Mix all ingredients together. Chill for 1 hour. Cover 4 cups of cooked brown rice with the lamb mixture. Garnish with red apples.

Variation:
Vinaigrette can be used instead of goat's yogurt and soy mayonnaise.

HOLIDAY RICE

1 onion
1 clove garlic
2 bacon rashers (optional)
1 cup chopped celery
½ cup pine nuts
3-4 cups cooked brown rice
1 cup shelled prawns/shrimps
1 cup chopped pineapple (optional)

In a large pan sauté onion, garlic, and bacon rashers until just cooked. Add chopped celery and pine nuts and sauté until pine nuts begin to brown. Add cooked brown rice, shelled prawns and chopped fresh pineapple. Heat through.

CHICKEN RICE SALAD

4 cups cooked rice
3 cups diced cooked chicken
1 cup sliced celery
1 cup orange or mandarin segments
good sprinkle of chopped mint
salt and pepper

Mix all ingredients together. Make a dressing of soy mayonnaise or vinaigrette and toss through the salad. Garnish with chopped capsicum, chives and toasted almonds.

TANGY RICE SALAD

1½ cups cooked brown rice
½ cup chopped celery
½ cup chopped cashews
1½ cups goats yogurt or 1 cup nut cream
2 tablespoons (1 oz/30 g) mango chutney

Mix together brown rice, chopped celery, chopped cashews, goat's yogurt or nut cream and mango chutney. Serve with sliced beetroot and cucumber vinaigrette.

INDIAN RICE

1 tablespoon (20 ml/¾ fl oz) non-dairy margarine or oil
1 tablespoon (½ oz/15 g) curry powder
½ cup mixed cashews and raisins
1 sliced onion
1 apple, cored and diced
2½ cups cooked brown rice

Sauté mixed cashews and raisins, sliced onion and apple in margarine or oil. Add curry powder. Add cooked brown rice and season. Heat through. Serve with green peas.

SWEET SESAME RICE

1 onion
1 red pepper (optional)
1 cup (155 g/5 oz) mixed dried fruit
½ cup chopped nuts
½ cup ground sesame seeds
¼-½ teaspoon ground cloves
salt (to taste)
3 cups cooked brown rice

Sauté until golden: onion, red pepper, chopped mixed dried fruits, chopped nuts, and ground sesame seeds. When cooked stir in ground cloves, and cooked brown rice. Heat through. Serve with steamed greens.

RICE PILAU

2 cups brown rice
1.25 litres/2 pints chicken stock
1 tablespoon oil
½ teaspoon allspice
1 small onion
1 clove garlic
½ teaspoon grated ginger
⅓ teaspoon garam marsala
2 cardamon pods
1 stick cinnamon
1 bay leaf
4 tablespoons (15 g/½ oz) chopped almonds
½ cup (90 g/3 oz) raisins
2 tablespoons (40 ml/1¼ fl oz) rose water (optional)

In an oven proof dish, fry onion, garlic and ginger lightly in oil. Add rice, stock, spices and mix well. Cover and bake at 180°C/350°F/Gas 4, for approximately 1 hour. Stir in raisins, and rose water after 45 minutes cooking. Stir again before serving. Garnish with chopped almonds.

CHINESE RICE

1 large onion
1-2 cups chopped vegetables (eg carrots, mushrooms, celery, bean sprouts)
3 cups cooked brown rice
1 cup pre-cooked beans (eg soy)
2 tablespoons (40 ml/1¼ fl oz) tamari soy sauce
toasted seeds and nuts

In a large oiled pan or wok, sauté onion and chopped vegetables quickly, giving the carrots, etc a little longer. Add brown rice and heat through. Add pre-cooked beans and tamari soy sauce. Heat through and garnish with toasted seeds and nuts (eg sunflower, sesame.)

VEGETABLE KEBABS WITH JAVA RICE

1 green pepper/capsicum
1 red pepper/capsicum
250 g/8 oz green zucchini/courgettes
250 g/8 oz yellow zucchini/courgettes
250 g/8 oz button mushrooms
½ cauliflower
4 onions
MARINADE:
½ cup soy sauce
1 cup water
2 tablespoons lemon juice
½ teaspoon grated green ginger
2 cloves garlic
2 teaspoons curry powder (or to taste)
RICE:
1½ cups (280 g/9 oz) long grain brown rice
1 onion
1 clove garlic
½ teaspoon grated green ginger
2 tablespoons oil
¼ cup chopped almonds
½ cup (175 g/2½ oz) currants
⅓ cup (60 g/2 oz) chutney
pinch tumeric

Divide cauliflower into small flowerettes. Soak in cold salted water for 30 minutes. Drain. Cook in boiling salted water for 5 minutes. Drain. Combine soy sauce, peeled crushed garlic, water, curry powder, ginger and lemon juice in a large bowl. Add peppers cut into 2.5 cm/1" squares and zucchini cut diagonally into slices, mushrooms with stems removed, drained cauliflower and peeled onions cut into squares. Toss well. Stand at room temperature for 1 hour. Thread vegetables onto skewers. Place onto oven trays, grill/broil under moderate heat 8-10 minutes, brushing occasionally with remaining marinade. Serve on bed of rice. Remove skewers if desired.

RICE

Cook rice uncovered in boiling salted water 20-30 minutes, drain.
Heat oil in a pan. Add crushed garlic. Cook until garlic just changes
colour. Add peeled chopped onion, turmeric and ginger. Cook 2
minutes longer. Add currants, chutney, almonds and rice. Stir well
and continue to cook a few minutes longer until rice is heated
through.

DESSERT RICE

1½ cups cooked brown rice
½ cup toasted ground sesame seeds
½ cup honey
½ cup coconut
1 cup pineapple pieces
1 banana
½-1 cup other fruit as desired
1 cup light nut cream or goat's yogurt
chopped nuts for garnish

Mix all ingredients together. Sprinkle with chopped nuts.

MAIN COURSES

GREEK BAKED FISH

1 whole fish, approximately 1½ kg/3 lb eg snapper/sea bass/bream
small handful parsley, chopped
brown rice, cooked
rice bran
4-5 gloves garlic
¾ cup/190 ml oil (olive oil plus safflower oil or substitute)
½ kg/1 lb chopped tomatoes

Stuff fish with mixture of cooked rice, rice bran, parsley, salt and pepper. In a small pan sauté 4-5 cloves garlic in oil until golden. Add three quarters of a cup of oil (half olive, half safflower) and 1 lb/500 g chopped tomatoes and simmer for ten minutes. Pour this mixture over fish and bake at 180°C/350°F/Gas 4, for approximately 30 minutes, depending on size of the fish. Serve with brown rice and green vegetables or a Greek salad.

MIDDLE EASTERN STUFFED FISH

1 whole fish, about 1½ g/3 lb
1 large ripe tomato
3 tablespoons (60 ml/2 fl oz) oil
125 g/¼ lb almonds, chopped
4 tablespoons (80 ml/2½ fl oz) lemon juice
6 prunes, stoned and chopped
125 g/¼ lb sultanas/seedless raisins
4-5 sprigs parsley, chopped

Clean fish and salt inside if desired. Mix together the almonds, lemon juice, prunes, sultanas and parsley and stuff mixture into fish cavity. Secure with toothpicks. Chop tomato and mix with the oil. Cook tomato and oil mixture for 5 minutes on top of the stove. Pour mixture over fish and bake in a moderate oven (180°C/350°F/Gas 4) for 30 minutes.

GINGER SNAPPER/SEA BASS

1 snapper, approximately 1½ kg/3 lb.

Stuff the snapper with a mixture of fried bacon, cooked rice, shallots, tumeric, capsicum, oil, egg or similar suitable combination, according to the rotation plan. Cover with foil and bake for 45 minutes in a moderate oven (180°C/350°F/Gas 4) and cover with ginger sauce during cooking.

GINGER SAUCE:
2 cups chicken or fish stock
2 tablespoons (22 g/¾ oz) cornflour/cornstarch or substitute
4 pieces of ginger, peeled & grated
2 tablespoons (40 ml/1¼ fl oz) tamari
1 teaspoon/5 g sugar
1 tablespoon (20 ml/¾ fl oz) dry sherry

Combine all ingredients in a saucepan. Heat, stirring constantly until the sauce thickens. Reduce the heat and simmer for 2-3 minutes. The sauce may be strained to remove the ginger.

MEDITERRANEAN STYLE MULLET

4 mullet
flour of choice
olive oil
½ kg/1 lb tomatoes
1 large clove garlic, crushed
salt and pepper
stuffed olives
anchovy fillets
lemon

Coat fish lightly with seasoned flour. Fry in hot olive oil, turning once and keep warm. Chop tomatoes and stew them until soft in a little olive oil with the garlic. Season and rub through a sieve (or blender). Arrange fish on dish, pour over the tomato purée, garnish with olives and anchovy fillets.

TEMPURA

choose a selection of vegetables—carrot, pumpkin, broccoli, cauliflower, onion etc.
cubes of fish or other seafood of your choice—prawns/shrimps, scallops etc.
oil for deep frying
flour for coating
egg white if allowed

Coat vegetables and fish lightly in flour, beaten egg if allowed and again flour. Deep fry all ingredients till golden brown. Serve immediately with a sauce of ½ tamari, ½ water and grated ginger to taste.

Variation:
Whitebait—small whole fish about 5 cm/2 inches long; usually available at fish markets. They can be similarly prepared and individually deep fried. Serve with tomato, vinegared salad and/or mashed potato.

STEAMED CALAMARI

½ kg/1 lb calamari, cleaned and cut into strips
small handful chopped parsley
1 clove garlic, minced
½ teaspoon ground cumin (optional)
juice of 1 lemon
2 tablespoons (40 ml/1¼ fl oz) olive oil

Simmer all ingredients except lemon juice in a lightly covered pan. When the calamari begins to steam, add the lemon juice and cook a further 15-20 minutes.

FISH RISSOLES

potatoes and pumpkin cooked and mashed, or leftovers
small can drained salmon, mackerel or sardines
onion flakes or fresh onion, chives and herbs to taste
maize meal or substitute
oil for frying

Mash all ingredients together. The mixture should be stiff. Do not add butter or oil. Form the mix into patties, roll in maize meal and fry lightly in oil or margarine; or bake 20-30 minutes at 180°C/350°F/Gas 4. Serve with tomato sauce or a substitute.

DELICIOUS RISSOLES

2 cups cooked brown rice
1 large tin drained mackerel
⅓ cup rice bran
1 small onion
1 grated carrot
½ cup (60 g/2 oz) ground raw cashews

Mix together to form patties. Can be fried lightly in oil or margarine or baked 20-30 minutes in a moderate oven 180°C/350°F/Gas 4.

PAUL'S FAVOURITE TUNA DISH

oil
cornflour/cornstarch
onion
1 cup (250 ml/8 fl oz) coconut milk
1 cup water
1 can tuna
vegetables or other leftovers, diced
curry to taste
salt
pepper

Heat oil, stir in cornflour, blend in milk, water and stir. Add onion, curry, seasoning and vegetables. Simmer until mixture thickens to the consistency of thick cream. Add tuna and heat through. Serve on a bed of rice.

TUNA RICE CAKES

180 g can/6 oz tuna, drained and flaked
1½ cups cooked brown rice
2 large sticks of celery, finely chopped
1 large onion, finely chopped
¼ cup (30 g/1 oz) rice flour
3 eggs separated

Combine tuna, rice, celery, onion, flour and egg yolks. Mix well. Beat egg whites until stiff but not dry. Fold into tuna mix. Drop mixture by ¼ cupfuls into a hot pan which has been slightly oiled. Cook, turning once until golden brown on both sides.

GEMFISH/SEA PIKE/BARRACUDA WITH BITE

4 gemfish (or substitute)
2 tablespoons (40 ml/1¼ fl oz) non-dairy margarine or oil
salt and pepper

1 orange
1 lemon

Place fish in greased baking dish, season with salt and pepper and dot with small pieces of margarine or oil. Cut orange and lemon in half. Juice one half of each and pour half of this mixture over the fish. Place fish under a high grill/broiler for about 4 minutes. Slice remaining fruit, top fish with sliced fruit and remaining juice. Return to grill and cook a further 4 minutes. Remove fish when golden. Serve with greens of your choice and mashed potato, or make mock mashed potato out of well-cooked millet.

BLENDER FISH CURRY

½ kg/1 lb fish cutlets or fillets
2 tablespoons ground coriander
¾ teaspoon ground fennel
¼ teaspoon cumin
½ teaspoon tumeric
1 large onion, grated
1 clove garlic, crushed
1 teaspoon finely chopped green ginger
1 cup (250 ml/8 fl oz) thick coconut milk
1 stalk lemon grass
lemon juice to taste (1 tablespoon)

Blend all ingredients, except the lemon grass and fish. Pour into a large pot or frying pan—bring to the boil. Add lemon grass and simmer for 10 minutes. Arrange fish in pan and cook over low heat for 10 minutes or until tender.

COCONUT MILK:
2 cups (185 g/6 oz) dessicated/shredded coconut into a bowl, add 2½ cups (625 ml/1 pt) hot water, let cool, knead with hands and strain, squeezing out most of the juice. Repeat for thinner milk.

SEAFOOD KEBABS

squares of firm fish
whole king prawns/shrimps
wedges of onions
wedges of tomatoes
wedges of capsicum/red or green peppers
whole mushrooms

Thread onto wooden skewers, basting generously with oil and tamari soy sauce. Barbecue or grill/broil. Serve on rice.

SCAMPI

500 g/1 lb raw king prawns/shrimps
rice bran
corn meal or substitute
oil
garlic to taste
oregano to taste

Arrange prawns on a baking dish. Cover with a mixture of rice bran, corn meal or substitute, oil, garlic and oregano. Bake 20 minutes at 350°F/180°C/Gas 4 (moderate oven).

COLD SAVOURY CALAMARI

500 g/1 lb cleaned squid
½ cup lemon juice
⅓ cup (85 ml/2½ fl oz) oil
1 clove garlic
good pinch chopped parsley

Cut squid into narrow rings, about 5 mm/¼ inch wide. Drop into boiling water, then simmer 10-15 minutes, or until tender. Drain. Combine lemon juice, oil and squid, cover. Refrigerate overnight. 2 hours before use, add crushed garlic and parsley to marinade. Mix well.

STIR-FRIED FISH

1 kg/2 lbs firm fish pieces
zucchini slices/courgettes
mushroom slices
bean sprouts
broccoli
2 cloves garlic
1 onion
fresh ginger to taste
tamari sauce (soy sauce)
lemon juice

In a wok or fry-pan sauté garlic, onion, pieces of ginger and pieces of fish. After a couple of minutes, stirring, add broccoli flowerettes, slices of zucchini, mushroom and finally bean sprouts. Season with tamari soy sauce and lemon juice. Serve with brown rice.

SEAFOOD STEW

3 fresh ripe tomatoes, peeled (or 1 can tomatoes)
½ cup stock, fish or vegetable
150 g scallops
150 g green prawns/shrimps
500 g/1 lb fish pieces, preferably boneless
salt and pepper
1 clove garlic, crushed
1 teaspoon curry powder
1 tablespoon currants
piece orange rind
¼ cup (45 g/1½ oz) coconut or 2 tablespoons coconut cream
2 teaspoons vinegar
1 teaspoon sugar

Sauté garlic in oil. Simmer all ingredients except seafood, for ½ hour to create a sauce. When ready to eat, cook seafood lightly in sauce (about 5 minutes). Serve with brown rice and greens or salad.

MACROBIOTIC STOCKPOT

1 chicken carcass
½ cup brown rice
1½ litres/2⅔ pts water
1 stalk celery, chopped
¾ cup (20g/⅔ oz) dried Japanese mushrooms
¼ cup (10 g/⅓ oz) hijike seaweed
1 tablespoon miso paste

Combine first four ingredients. Bring to boil and simmer approximately 1 hour. Remove carcass and return any chicken pieces to soup. Soak mushrooms and hijike for ½ hour in cold water. Add these to soup and cook a further ½ hour. Before serving stir in miso paste, thinned with a little soup. Do not boil miso.

Variations:
Substitute other seaweeds, eg wakame.
Add soba (buckwheat noodles).

CASHEW CHICKEN

1½ kg/3 lbs chicken (approximately 8 pieces)
¼ cup (60 ml/2 fl oz) vegetable oil
2 onions finely chopped
½ cup (125 ml/4 fl oz) chicken stock
½ cup coconut milk (fresh if possible)
4 whole cloves
1 cup (125 g/4 oz) coarsely chopped unsalted roasted cashews
2 tablespoons (30 ml/1 fl oz) fresh lime juice, or lemon juice
freshly ground black pepper to taste

Dry chicken. Brown chicken evenly in oil over moderate heat. Transfer to a dish. Pour off excess fat. Add onions to pan and cook about 5 minutes, stirring frequently, until translucent. Add chicken stock, coconut milk and cloves and stirring constantly, bring to a simmer over moderate heat. Return chicken and juices to the sauce and cook very slowly, partially covered for about 30 minutes, until chicken is cooked. Transfer chicken to a plate and keep warm. Sieve cooking liquid, taking out cloves. Blend in onion. There should be about 1 cup of sauce. Add more chicken stock or water if necessary. Simmer in pan, stirring, add cashews, lime/lemon juice and pepper. Add chicken to warm and serve accompanied with brown rice, and vegetables of choice.

BRAISED CHICKEN AND MUSHROOMS

300 g/9½ oz raw chicken meat
1 level tablespoon (10 g/⅓ oz) cornflour/cornstarch
1 egg white
1 tablespoon (20 ml/⅛ fl oz) tamari soy sauce
2 tablespoons (40 ml/¼ fl oz) oil
5-6 fresh mushrooms (or dried mushrooms soaked in warm water)
1 small piece of green ginger cut finely
1 stalk celery, sliced diagonally
¼ cup water
few drops sesame oil
1 tablespoon (20 ml/⅔ fl oz) dry sherry
2 teaspoons/5 g cornflour/cornstarch extra

Cut chicken into thin strips. Combine cornflour, egg white and tamari and coat chicken well. Heat oil, sauté chicken until brown. Remove and drain. Slice mushrooms. Add extra oil if necessary. Fry mushrooms, ginger and celery for a few minutes. Add water and sesame oil and allow it to boil. Add sherry, return chicken to pan, simmer with lid on for 5 minutes. Remove lid, cook until chicken is tender. Thicken with cornflour blended in a small amount of water.

CHICKEN 'N LENTIL BALLS

¾ cup lentils (cooked)
4 cups hot water or stock
500 g/1 lb chicken, finely chopped
1 teaspoon salt
freshly ground black pepper to taste

1 egg
cornflour/cornstarch
Drain lentils. Combine with chicken, seasonings and egg. Mix well. Shape into balls. Toss in cornflour. Deep fry in hot oil for 10-15 minutes or until golden brown.

ROAST DUCK

1½ kg/3 lb duck
oil for basting
rosemary and sage
Tie duck's legs together and wings to breast with string. Dust duck with rosemary and sage. Bake in moderate oven on wire rack in baking dish for 20 minutes, breast side up. Remove duck and prick all over then return for further 20 minutes, breast side down. Cook a further 20 minutes, breast side up.

SAUTÉED LIVER

500 g/1 lb liver, sliced thin, coated with rice flour
1 clove garlic
1 onion
mushrooms
4 shallots
tamari soy sauce
Heat 2 tablespoons oil in a pan and brown liver quickly with chopped garlic. Add finely sliced onion, a handful of mushrooms, and cook until meat is evenly browned. Add 4 chopped shallots, and tamari to taste. Continue cooking, stirring constantly for approximately 10 minutes.

LAMB'S FRY WITH PEPPERCORNS

1 lambs fry/liver
2 tablespoons (40 ml/¼ fl oz) oil
salt
parsley
1 tablespoon (8 g/¼ oz) whole black peppercorns, ground with mortar and pestle

Cut liver into strips about 1 cm/½" thick. Sprinkle strips with peppercorns until well-coated. Heat oil in frying pan and cook liver quickly, turning gently until lightly browned on all sides. This takes little more than 3 minutes. Transfer to heated serving plate and sprinkle with salt and parsley. Serve with salad and chips. Omit peppercorns for children.

LAMB CASSEROLE

8 lamb chops
2 onions
125 g/4 oz bacon
60 g/2 oz mushrooms
1 bulb fennel
3 cloves garlic
60 g/2 oz butter, or oil for sautéeing
¾ cup (125 ml/6 fl oz) dry white wine
1 cup water
1 tablespoon (10 g/⅓ oz) tomato paste
salt, pepper
2 tablespoons (200 g/⅔ oz) potato flour, cornflour or arrowroot
2 tablespoons (20 ml/⅔ fl oz) water extra

Melt butter in pan, add chops and brown well on both sides. Remove from pan and place in ovenproof dish in one layer. Add to pan quartered onions, crushed garlic, sliced fennel and bacon pieces and sliced mushrooms. Cook for 2 minutes. Add wine, water and tomato paste, bring to boil, remove from heat and season well with salt and pepper. Pour vegetable mixture over chops, cover and bake in moderate oven for 45 minutes or until chops are tender. Remove chops and keep warm. Pour sauce and vegetables into saucepan. Combine flour and extra water. Pour into sauce. Stir until boiling. Pour over chops

Variation

Substitute veal chops for lamb chops.

HUNGARIAN GOULASH

1 kg/2 lbs steak, cubed
rice flour
130 g/4 oz bacon (optional) chopped
1 clove garlic chopped
2 large onions chopped
2 tablespoons sweet paprika
¼ teaspoon caraway seeds
1 large tomato, chopped
1 green pepper/capsicum, chopped
1 hot pepper (optional)
4 cups water
salt
pepper
parsley

Lightly coat meat with flour. In large frypan, fry bacon, mix in garlic, onions, paprika, caraway seeds, tomato, green and hot peppers, and sauté until vegetables are tender. Add meat and continue cooking for another 5 minutes. Blend in water, salt and pepper, cover pan and cook gently for another 1 to 1½ hours or until beef is tender. Sprinkle with paprika and parsley. Serve with soy noodles or brown rice.

JAPANESE BUCKWHEAT GRIDDLECAKES

1½ cups (185 g/6 oz) buckwheat flour
⅔ cups (170 ml/5 fl oz) chicken stock
pinch salt
½ teaspoon baking powder
200 g/6½ oz cabbage
100 g/3½ oz beef
prawns/shrimps
pork or other protein
4 eggs
4 mushrooms (optional)
vegetable oil for hot plate

In large bowl sift together flour, salt and baking powder. Gradually add soup stock. Shred cabbage and chop meat into small pices. Mix together 1 egg, quarter each of the dough, cabbage and meat. Spoon mixture onto hot plate of griddle iron, or into well oiled frypan. When about 60% cooked, turn over. When cooked through, turn again and top with soy sauce, or the traditional Japanese garnishes, such as dried seaweed or bonito (small dried fish).

OXTAIL STEW

1 oxtail
1½ cups water
1 tablespoon oil
salt and pepper
tamari soy sauce
1 carrot
1 turnip
1 onion
½ lemon
cornflour/cornstarch (or substitute)

Cut tail into 5 cm/2" chunks and trim fat. Heat oil in pan and brown meat. Add water and cubed vegetables. Pressure cook for 35 minutes. Before serving, thicken stew with cornflour, tamari and lemon juice mixture. If pressure cooker unavailable, simmer in a large pot, adding more water as required.

OSSO BUCCO

4 veal knuckles/leg (ask your butcher to cut)
90 g/3 oz margarine or substitute oil
2 carrots chopped
2 large onions finely chopped
3 sticks celery finely chopped
2 cloves garlic
flour (what you can have)
salt
pepper
2 tablespoons oil
2 x 400 g/13 oz cans whole tomatoes
½ cup (125 ml/4 fl oz) dry red wine, or sherry mixed with water
2 cups (500 ml/6 fl oz) beef stock
1 teaspoon basil
1 teaspoon thyme
1 bayleaf
2.5 cm/1" strip lemon rind
1 teaspoon grated lemon rind
small handful chopped parsley

Sauté carrots, onions, celery and one crushed garlic clove in a small amount of margarine or oil. Cook gently until the onions are golden brown. Transfer to a large baking dish. Coat shanks with flour seasoned with salt and pepper. Heat remaining margarine or oil in large frying pan, add shanks, brown well on all sides. Pack shanks on top of vegetables. Purée tomatoes. Drain fat from pan in which veal was cooked. Add wine, beef stock, tomatoes, basil, thyme, bayleaf and a strip of lemon rind. Bring sauce to boil, season with salt and pepper. Pour sauce over veal shanks. Cover casserole, bake in moderate oven until cooked approximately 1½ hours, stirring occasionally. Garnish with a mixture of crushed garlic, chopped parsley and grated lemon rind.

GOURMET POTATOES

6 large potatoes
750 g/1½ lb choice mince/ground meat
1 onion, finely chopped
salt
1 teaspoon rosemary
1 egg (optional)
¼ teaspoon tabasco
1 tablespoon (15 g/½ oz) curry powder

Bake potatoes in a moderate oven until cooked through. Cool, until easy to handle. Cut top off each potato and scoop out the middle with a teaspoon. Combine potato flesh with other ingredients and mix well. Stuff potato shells with a mixture and bake in a moderate oven for about 40 minutes, or until toasted on top.

STUFFED TOMATOES

6 large tomatoes
1½ cups (210 g/6¾ oz) cooked brown rice
3 anchovies, mashed
black pepper to taste
sprinkle chopped parsley

Remove pulp from the tomatoes. In a pan combine the oil, tomato pulp, anchovies, sugar and pepper. Cook for 10 minutes, stirring occasionally. Add the rice and parsley and mix well. Fill the tomatoes with the mixture and bake in a greased dish for 15 minutes in a moderate oven.

LAMB SHISH KEBAB

1 kg/2 lbs lean boneless lamb cubes
1 large firm tomato
1 large green pepper
vegetable salt to taste
freshly ground black pepper to taste

If time allows, presoak the lamb for at least 2 hours in a marinade of 1 part olive oil and 2 parts lemon juice, plus 1 chopped onion. Turn occasionally. Preheat grill/broiler and thread the lamb cubes on 4 long skewers. Thread vegetables on separate skewers as they take less time to cook. Brush meat with marinade juices, or oil and lemon juice and grill about 10 cm/4" from the heat, turning the skewers occasionally until the vegetables brown and the lamb is done to personal taste. (Pink lamb — 10 minutes, well done lamb — 15 minutes). Serve with steamed rice or tabouli.

Variation:

Chicken fillet and chicken liver kebabs. Make a more exotic marinade by adding 1 teaspoon cumin, 1 teaspoon paprika and 1 teaspoon grated ginger. In this case, omit tomato and combine meat and vegetables on this same skewer.

SAUTÉED BRAINS

3-4 sets brains
2 cloves garlic (or to taste)
oil
½ cup rice bran, corn meal or substitute
salt and pepper
parsley

Simmer brains in water to cover, about 20 minutes. Drain, cool slightly, and remove membranes. Cut into ¼"/1 cm strips, coat in rice bran and fry until golden on both sides. Add garlic, either to simmering water or to oil before frying. Season and garnish with parsley. May be served also as a starter or breakfast dish.

HONEY GLAZED PORK CHOPS

1½ kg/3 lbs pork chops
½ teaspoon salt
pinch five spice powder
1 teaspoon salt, extra

2 tablespoons oil
⅓ cup honey
1½ tablespoons (30 ml/1 fl oz) tamari soy sauce
⅓ cup (85 ml/2½ fl oz) orange juice
1 teaspoon grated green ginger
1 teaspoon cornflour/cornstarch or substitute
2 tablespoons water

Sprinkle chops with 5 spice powder and place in baking dish. Pour combined honey, soy sauce, orange juice and ginger over chops. Bake for 45 minutes, spooning sauce over occasionally until cooked through. Remove pork from the baking dish and keep warm. Strain pan juices into a small saucepan. Allow to stand a few minutes then skim off the fat. Add combined cornflour and water, mix well. Stir over medium heat until sauce boils and thickens. Serve with chops.

CHILI CON CARNE

1 onion, chopped
1 clove garlic, crushed
½ kg/1 lb choice minced/ground beef
2 cups (220 g/7 oz) cooked red beans (kidney, aduki)
1 can tomatoes or
2 large fresh tomatoes
1 teaspoon chili powder or to taste

Brown onion and garlic. Add chili powder with meat and brown well. Add tomatoes and simmer for 20 minutes. Add cooked beans and simmer further 15 minutes before serving. Serve with brown rice and greens.

Italian Variation:
Bolognaise sauce—Omit chili and beans; substitute oregano and vegetables. Serve with 100% buckwheat noodles.

Mexican Variation:
Serve with taco shells, shredded lettuce, tomato cubes and sprouts. Include (or disguise) more vegetables—e.g. carrot, peas, green beans, turnips, parsnips etc.

SPINACH PIE

CRUST:
Mix with fork ½ cup (60 g/2 oz) barley flour, 1 tablespoon oil and a pinch of salt. Add enough cold water to barely bind the mixture. Form into a ball and refrigerate for at least half an hour. Thinly roll. (See baking section for alternative pie crusts)

FILLING:
2 cups cooked spinach/spring or collard greens
½ cup (60 g/2 oz) ground nuts
1 chopped onion
1 clove garlic, chopped
1 or 2 eggs
salt and pepper
pinch of nutmeg

Mix all ingredients and place in partially cooked crust. Bake at 180°C/350°F/Gas 4 (moderate oven) for 35-40 minutes. Serve with brown rice and salad.

STEAK AND KIDNEY PIE

Adapt favourite recipe but do not thicken with flour. As an alternative, simmer garlic, onions, steak, kidney, mushrooms and tomato until a sauce forms. Crustless pies are suitable. Top with mashed pumpkin as an alternative to mashed potato.

BUTTER BEAN RISSOLES

1 kg/2 lbs mashed beans
small handful parsley, chopped
half an onion, finely chopped
2 tablespoons (15 g/½ oz) ground nuts
1 beaten egg
herbs etc

Combine all ingredients. Shape into rissoles. Fry in oil for about 5 minutes each side.

Variation:
Add mashed pumpkin and cook as a loaf, sprinkled with maize meal or substitute and dot with margarine. Bake at 180°C/350°F/Gas 4 (moderate oven) until heated through.

RICE AND LENTIL RISSOLES

1½ cups (210 g/6¾ oz) brown rice, cooked
¾ cup (155 g/5 oz) cooked lentils
4 shallots, finely chopped
2 tablespoons (15 g/½ oz) toasted sesame seeds
Mix the rice, lentils and shallots into small rissoles. Roll each rissole in sesame seeds. May be warmed through in the oven or eaten cold.

NUTLOAF

2 cups (250 g/8 oz) ground nuts, or seeds, or mixture of both
1 chopped onion
3 cloves garlic
3 stalks celery
2 eggs
½ cup (90 g/3 oz) rice bran
1 cup (120 g/4½ oz) cooked rice
1 tablespoon (20 ml/⅔ fl oz) tamari
fresh herbs to taste
Mix all the ingredients and bake for 40 minutes as 180°C/350°F/Gas 4.

BEANS IN TOMATO SAUCE

1 kg/2 lbs dried borlotti beans
30 g/1 oz margarine
1 clove garlic
2 onions
45 g/1½ oz can anchovy fillets

3 tomatoes
1½ tablespoons (15 g/½ oz) tomato paste
1 teaspoon basil
½ teaspoon sugar
1 cup water
salt
pepper

Soak the beans overnight. Finely crush the garlic. Peel and finely chop onions. Drain and finely chop anchovy fillets. Peel and chop the tomatoes. Melt the margarine in a saucepan, add garlic, anchovies, onion and tomato. Cook until the onion is transparent. Add tomato paste, basil, sugar and beans, mix well until combined, Add water, bring to boil for 3 minutes, reduce heat, simmer covered for 30 minutes or until the beans are tender. Season with salt and pepper.

Variation:
Use other types of beans, especially kidney beans and great northern beans. These may require longer cooking.

BABY LIMA SPECIAL

2 onions
2 cloves garlic
250 g/8 oz mushrooms
mustard
2 cups cooked baby lima beans

Sauté onions and garlic in oil. Add mustard to taste and chopped mushrooms. Stir in baby lima beans. Add a little liquid and allow to simmer for ten minutes. Thicker sauce may be obtained by mashing some of the beans.

CURRIED LENTILS

Make a favourite curry using lentils instead of meat. Serve on brown rice with side dishes like cucumber/goat's yogurt, tomato/onion, banana/coconut. See recipe for Blender Fish Curry.

RAW RISSOLES

125 g/4 oz ground seeds (sesame, sunflower, pumpkin)
125 g/4 oz ground nuts (cashew, almond, etc)
1 tablespoon flour
⅓ cup (85 ml/2½ fl oz) goat's yogurt or 2 eggs
1 grated carrot
1 teaspoon lemon juice
chives
parsley and/or tamari soy sauce for flavour. (This mixture may be kept a couple of days in the refrigerator.)

Mix the ingredients together and press into rissoles.

MILLET CASSEROLE

225 g/7 oz millet
1 litre/1¾ pts stock
2 tablespoons (40 ml/1¼ fl oz) oil
1 carrot, chopped
2 onions, chopped
1 cup (90 g/3 oz) sliced mushrooms
2 cloves garlic
tamari

Brown the millet in a frypan. Using a large casserole dish, fry garlic and onions on top of the stove until lightly browned. Add browned millet, carrots, stock and tamari, stir to combine and bake in a moderate oven (180°C/350°F/Gas 4) tightly covered for about 2 hours or until the millet is tender.

DESSERTS

A different stewed fruit   *174*
Apple sauce uncooked   *179*
Apricot sorbet   *176*
Baked apples   *176*
Baked pears   *180*
Basic agar jelly/gelatin recipe   *178*
Carob gelato   *179*
Carob jelly/gelatin   *176*
Delicious rhubarb   *174*
Fruit and nut crumble   *175*
Hot barley dessert   *174*
Hot fruit salad   *177*
Icy poles   *177*
Lemon sago   *173*
Mango sorbet   *177*
Orange egg cream   *173*
Orange sherbet   *180*
Passionfruit flummery   *178*
Rice and raisin pudding   *180*
Rice berry pudding   *172*
Stewed quinces   *175*
Super prune whip   *173*
Sweet potato sorbet   *178*
Tofu strawberry whip   *181*

RICE BERRY PUDDING

1 cup cooked brown rice
1 cup nut milk
2 eggs
1-2 tablespoons honey
vanilla (optional)

1 cup fresh or frozen berries (such as raspberries, blueberries blackberries, etc)
OR
1 cup dried fruit (eg sultanas/seedless raisin, chopped dates etc).
Combine rice, milk, eggs and honey in a saucepan and stir over low heat until thick. Add fruit.

LEMON SAGO

2 cups sago
2 cups water (add more if too thick)
2 lemons
1 orange (optional)
1 banana
2 tablespoons honey or to taste
Bring slowly to the boil, stirring constantly. Simmer until thick.

ORANGE EGG CREAM

1 tablespoon (15 g/½ oz) gelatin dissolved in ½ cup hot water
1 cup orange juice
1 teaspoon lemon juice
2 tablespoons honey
2 beaten egg yolks
2 egg whites
Beat egg whites until stiff. Mix other ingredients and gently fold in egg whites. Set in refrigerator.

SUPER PRUNE WHIP

1 cup prunes, stewed and stoned
3 ripe bananas
1 apple (optional)
½ teaspoon almond extract
⅓ cup dessicated/shredded coconut
Blend all ingredients except coconut. Stir in coconut if desired.

DELICIOUS RHUBARB

½ bunch rhubarb cut in small cubes
½ cup raisins
½ cup dates
1 orange
1 litre/1¾ pts boiling water
¼ teaspoon salt
¼ teaspoon cayenne

Combine all ingredients. Bring to the boil and simmer for about 5 minutes. Pour into a bowl and allow to stand overnight in a cool place

HOT BARLEY DESSERT

barley
dried apricots
coconut
water

Cook soaked barley with chopped dried apricots or other dried fruit to taste. Towards the end of cooking stir in some coconut. Cooking takes at least half an hour. Leftovers make good breakfast with nutcream or goat's yogurt.

A DIFFERENT STEWED FRUIT

1 pineapple
2 kg/4 lb pears
500 g/1 lb prunes (optional)
500 ml/16 fl oz water
2 tablespoons (15 g/½ oz) arrowroot
slivered almonds (garnish)

Peel pineapple and cut into small pieces. Wash pears, core and cut into wedges. Add prunes, water and dissolved arrowroot. Bring to the boil and simmer for about 10 minutes. Cool and store in refrigerator, or freeze. Serve with slivered almonds sprinkled over top.

Variation:
Can be used as a base for crumble or pie.

STEWED QUINCES

½ kg/1 lb quinces
1 tablespoon honey (or to taste)
½ teaspoon cinnamon
½ teaspoon nutmeg
½ teaspoon cold pressed oil (milk tasting variety, apricot kernel or almond oil)

Boil quinces whole until soft. When cool, purée with honey, cinnamon, nutmeg and oil.

FRUIT AND NUT CRUMBLE

4 portions hot sweetened stewed fruit
1 tablespoon cooking oil
30 g/1 oz ground almonds
125 g/4 oz ground brown rice
25 g/¾ oz black sugar

Preheat oven to 200°C/400°F/Gas 6. Put fruit into an ovenproof dish and flatten the top evenly. Mix other ingredients and spoon evenly over stewed fruit. Leave a hole in the centre for the steam to escape. Bake 10-12 minutes. Serve hot or cold.

Variations:
Add or substitute sunflower seeds, sesame seeds, dates, coconut, etc.

BAKED APPLES

4 apples
dates
sultanas/seedless raisins
honey
nuts, seeds or coconut

Core a whole apple and pack your choice of chopped dried fruits, nuts and seeds into the hole. Drizzle a little honey (or substitute) on top. Bake 20-30 minutes (depending on size and type of apple), in a moderate oven (180°C/350°F/Gas 4). Serve plain or with nut cream or soy custard.

CAROB JELLY/GELATIN

1 cup warm water
1 teaspoon agar
3 tablespoons (100 ml/3 fl oz) honey
2 tablespoons (15 g/½ oz) carob
¼ cup sunflower oil
1 teaspoon vanilla

Dissolve agar in warm water. Blend all ingredients until smooth and pour into a mould or individual serving dishes. Chill.
Variation:
Add 1-2 eggs to final blend.

APRICOT SORBET

Fresh apricots
carrots
1-2 tablespoons fresh lemon juice

Prepare equal quantities of apricots and carrots. Gently stew apricots in water. Cook carrots until soft. Purée both in blender, add one or two tablespoons of fresh lemon juice, to taste. Put mixture into freezer trays — a shallow baking tin lined with foil works quite well —

and freeze for 2 to 3 hours. Stir the mixture every 30 minutes to break up the icy particles as they form. If this becomes too solid, removing from freezer in advance will allow it to soften again before serving.

Variation:
Substitute dried apricots, making up equal quantities of apricots and carrot purée.

ICY POLES

These can be made from fruit juices or diluted purées. Try adding coconut, grapes, chopped fruit, chopped nuts for variety. When making nut creams or butter in a blender there is no need to fiddle about trying to extract every last drop. Just add water, or diluted fruit juice, or some fresh fruit and water and whizz into a milky mixture for iceblocks. If on a rotation diet, label the blocks to show ingredients. Freezer labels work well.

MANGO SORBET

Purée the flesh of ripe mangoes and freeze. Sweet ripe mangoes need no additional ingredients. Freeze the mixture by putting into shallow trays and freeze for 2 to 3 hours. Stir the mixture every 30 minutes to break up the icy particles as they form. If this becomes too cold and solid, removing from the freezer in advance will allow it to soften again before serving.

HOT FRUIT SALAD

small packed of dried fruit salad mix, about 200 g/6½ oz or combination of your choice, including prunes, figs, apricots, pears, apples, raisins etc
juice of 1 lemon
juice of 2 oranges
1 tablespoon honey

Cover fruit in water and soak overnight. Combine all ingredients and simmer until fruit is soft and cooked. If too much liquid remains, remove fruit with a slotted spoon and boil to reduce liquid. Serve with nut cream, goat's yogurt, soy custard, or just sprinkle with coconuts or toasted almonds.

SWEET POTATO SORBET

3-4 sweet potatoes—yellow
juice of 1 lemon
shredded, dessicated or fresh coconut or fresh or chopped nuts.

Cook sweet potatoes in little water until soft, or roast whole in the oven. Remove skin. Blend the potato pulp and lemon juice, using some of the cooking water if required to make a smooth purée. Add nuts or coconut to taste. Freeze in a shallow tray for at least 2-3 hours. Stir the mixture every 30 minutes to break up the icy particles as they form. If this becomes too cold and solid, remove from the freezer in advance, allowing it to soften again before serving.

BASIC AGAR JELLY RECIPE

3 cups any liquid (fruit juice is excellent)
1½ (20 g/⅔ oz) tablespoons powdered agar

Cook and stir constantly over a low flame until dissolved. Strain and cool. Whole pieces of fruit may be added to the jelly while setting.

PASSIONFRUIT FLUMMERY

4-6 passionfruit
1 tablespoon (15 g/½ oz) gelatine or agar
½ cup cold water
2 tablespoons (30 g/1 oz) flour (whichever allowed)
½ cup sugar
½ cup orange juice

1 tablespoon (20 ml/⅔ fl oz) lemon juice
1 cup hot water
passionfruit to decorate (optional)
Halve passionfruit and remove pulp. Set aside. Soak gelatine in cold water. Combine flour and sugar in a saucepan, add enough orange juice to blend to a smooth paste. Add remaining orange juice, lemon juice and hot water. Bring to the boil, stirring until mixture thickens. Add soaked gelatine, stir until dissolved. Cool then transfer to a large bowl and chill until starting to set. Beat well until very thick and at least double in volume. Add passionfruit pulp, beat again. Turn into serving dishes and chill until set. Decorate with extra passionfruit pulp if desired.

APPLE SAUCE UNCOOKED

2 juicy apples (peel and grate)
½ cup nut cream
1 tablespoon honey (or less)
Combine ingredients. Pour over any fruit or cereal, rice etc.

CAROB GELATO

2 cups water
¼-½ cup maple syrup or honey
1 cup strong black carob drink
2 egg whites
Put water and syrup in a saucepan and bring to the boil. Reduce heat. Simmer uncovered for 10 minutes. Cool. Add carob and mix well. Pour mixture into icecream trays (or a suitable shallow tin or plastic container), freeze for approximately 1½ hours – or until mixture is just firm. Remove from the freezer. Turn mixture into a bowl and beat until smooth with a fork. Fold in firmly beaten egg whites, return to tray, freeze until firm. Serves 4.
Variation:
Orange ice: 600 mls/19 fl oz water, ¼ cup maple syrup, 300 mls/10

fl oz orange juice, juice of 1 lemon, 1 egg white. Prepare as above.
Strawberry Ice: 300 mls water, ¼ cup maple syrup, 2 cups strawberries puréed through seive, 2 tablespoons lemon juice, 1 egg white. Prepare as for Carob gelato.
Lemon Gelato: ½ cup lemon juice, ¼ cup honey, ½ cup white wine (or water), ½ cup water, 1 egg white. Prepare as for Carob gelato.

BAKED PEARS

Cut pears in half, and scoop out core. Mix small amounts of lemon juice, orange juice, honey and powdered ginger. Pour mixture into hollows. Bake at least 15 minutes at 180°C/350°F/Gas 4.

ORANGE SHERBET

1½ cups orange juice and pulp
2 teaspoons agar
1 cup honey
¼ cup cold water
2 cups boiling water
½ cup lemon juice
rind of 3 oranges grated
Mix orange juice and rind, lemon and honey together. Leave until a syrup forms. Dissolve agar in boiling water. Add to cold water and other ingredients. Cool until soft (about 1 hour). Beat cooled fruit mixture until creamy. Serve with nut cream.

RICE AND RAISIN PUDDING

1 cup brown rice
¼ cup honey
1 litre/1¾ pts soy bean milk
add a few raisins and a little lemon rind
Bake for about 2 hours. Stir frequently.

TOFU STRAWBERRY WHIP

1 packet tofu (220-250 g/7-8 oz)
2 cups fresh strawberries
2 tablespoons honey, maple syrup or rice syrup
1 teaspoon pure vanilla extract

Combine tofu, 1 cup strawberries, honey and vanilla in a liquidizer. Purée until smooth and creamy. Spoon into four custard cups and top each portion with 3-4 strawberries. Add ½ cup milk (soy or nut) and purée to make a refreshing and healthy milkshake.

Variation:
'Choc Tofu' Add 2 tablespoons (15 g/½ oz) carob instead of strawberries and a little more honey. Top with walnuts. Use these as pie fillings.

BAKED FOODS & SNACKS

POTATO BREAD

1 cup warm mashed potato
½ cup sugar
½ cup soy milk or substitute
½ cup potato flour
2 heaped teaspoons baking powder
pinch salt
Optional:
1 cup sultanas
1 teaspoon allspice
1 teaspoon cinnamon

Blend sugar into potato slowly. Beat into a creamy mixture. Sift all flours, baking powder and salt. Add alternately with milk, starting and finishing with flour. Beat for a few minutes. Spoon into greased bar tin. Bake in preheated oven 180°C/350°F for 1 hour.

COPHA BREAD

300 g/9½ oz potato flour
90 g/3 oz arrowroot flour
90 g/3 oz soya flour
½ teaspoon salt
420 mls/14 fl oz water
60 g/2 oz baking powder
30 g/1 oz sugar
30 g/1 oz copha (melted and cooled)
dairy free margarine for greasing

Sift all dry ingredients together twice, gradually adding water while mixing. Add copha last. Pour into greased loaf tins. Bake at 190°C for 30-40 minutes.
Variation:
Add chopped dates when mixing.

QUICK SOYA BREAD

1½ cups (185 g/6 oz) soya flour
1¼ cups (155 g/5 oz) cornflour or arrowroot
20 g/⅔ oz baking powder
1 teaspoon sugar
½ teaspoon salt
30 g/1 oz shortening
¾ cup soy milk or substitute
1 egg

Sieve the dry ingredients into a basin, rub in the shortening. Mix in egg and milk. Pour into a greased tin. Bake in a moderate oven (about 180°C/350°F/Gas 4) for about 45 minutes.

SWEET PUMPKIN BREAD

½ cup (60 g/2 oz) cornstarch, potato starch, soy flour or combination
1¼ cup rice flour
1 tablespoon baking powder
½ teaspoon bicarbonate soda/baking soda
1 teaspoon cinnamon
½ teaspoon nutmeg
1 cup (155 g/5 oz) cooked pumpkin
2 eggs
⅓ cup margarine (non dairy)
⅔ cup (125 g/4 oz) black sugar
¼ cup (30 g/1 oz) chopped walnuts
¼ cup (40 g/1¼ oz) currants or substitute

Cream sugar and shortening. Add pumpkin and eggs and mix well. Sift dry ingredients (except fruit & nuts), and gradually add dry ingredients to creamed mixture. Finally stir in fruit and nuts. Grease 2 small or 1 large bread tin. Cook small loaves approximately forty five minutes and large loaves approximately 1 hour at 180°C/350°F/Gas 4. Test with skewer. Cool 15 minutes in pan before removing.

RICE BREAD

250 g/8 oz rice flour
½ teaspoon cream of tartar
2 tablespoons oil
½ teaspoon salt
180 mls/6 fl. oz. water

Combine water and oil. Gradually stir into sifted dry ingredients. Bake in greased bread tin about 30 minutes at 190°C/375°F/Gas 5.

SWEET BUCKWHEAT BREAD

1½ cups buckwheat flour
1 tablespoon baking powder
3 eggs
½ cup honey
1 teaspoon pure vanilla
1 cup sunflower oil

Mix flour and baking powder in bowl. Blend other ingredients well. Mix thoroughly into flour mixture. Bake at 190°C/375°F/Gas 5 about 30 minutes.

HOT CROSS MUFFINS

2½ cups nutritious mix, eg 1 cup rice bran, ¾ cup potato starch,
¾ cup rice flour
2 tablespoons (40 ml/1¼ fl. oz.) oil or milk free margarine
2 tablespoons (30 g/1 oz) black sugar
1 cup water (nutmilk or goat's yogurt)
2 teaspoon baking powder
3 eggs, separated
½ cup sultanas/seedless raisins or currants

Beat eggs until stiff. Mix all other ingredients. Fold in egg whites, plus sultanas or currants. Fill patty tins or muffin tins. Cut corner from plastic bag, mix potato starch to paste and pipe a cross on top before cooking at 200°C/400°F for 12 minutes if being reheated; 15 minutes if eating immediately.

PLAIN RICE BISCUITS (SAVOURY)

3 cups brown rice flour
½ teaspoon salt
1½ tablespoon sesame oil
¾ cup water

Rub oil into rice flour mixed with salt. Gradually add water to form dough. Knead gently for a couple of minutes. Roll into a ball and flatten with a fork. Bake at 180°C/350°F/Gas 4 for 20-25 minutes.

TOPLESS PIE CRUST

1½ cups (185 g/6 oz) flour mixture—choice of soy, rice, potato, corn, marzipan meal, arrowroot
1 cup oil
¼ cup (60 ml/2 fl. oz) nut milk or soy milk
½ teaspoon salt

Combine dry ingredients and moist ingredients separately. Add moist ingredients to dry with a fork. Press into shape over base of pie tin. Add pie filling of your choice. Bake at 200°C/400°F for 15 minutes and then a further 30 minutes at 180°C/350°F or until filling is cooked.

Variation:

Increase mixture and crumble remainder on top of pie, or use fruit crumble mixture on top of pie. Include ½ cup ground nuts in flour mixture.

NUTTY PIE CRUSTS

Two cups of any ground nuts will fill a 25 cm/9½" pie tin. Press nut meal into place firmly with fingers. A little oil added will help thin out the nut meal. Fill pie and bake at 200°C/400°F/Gas 6 until crust is lightly browned (may take from 20 to 40 minutes).

PLAIN BUCKWHEAT BISCUITS (SAVOURY)

2 cups (250 g/8 oz) buckwheat flour
1 teaspoon salt
½ teaspoon ground cinnamon, or to taste
2 tablespoons sesame oil
1 cup water
Rub oil through sifted dry ingredients. Gradually add water to form a thick batter. Drop teaspoonsful onto biscuit tray and top with a piece of nut or dried fruit. Bake at 180°C/350°F/Gas 4 for 25 minutes.

CORNFLOUR CRISPS

60 g/2 oz non dairy margarine
1 beaten egg
60 g/2 oz coconut
60 g/2 oz sugar
90 g/3 oz cornflour
1 teaspoon pure vanilla essence
Cream margarine and sugar. Add beaten egg. Fold in cornflour and coconut. Flavour with vanilla. Drop in spoonfuls on greased tray. Bake at 190°C/375°F/Gas 5 for 10-15 minutes.

PIKELETS

1 cup cornmeal
½ cup soyflour
½ cup buckwheat flour
1 teaspoon baking powder or 2 eggs
½ cup coconut
vanilla

salt
water

Blend all ingredients with sufficient water to form a very thick paste. Grease pan well. Cook small amounts and turn to brown both sides.
Variation:
Vary flours according to rotation plan.

APRICOT DELIGHTS

250 g/8 oz dried apricots
1 cup boiling water
2 tablespoons sesame seeds, toasted
½ cup (45 g/1½ oz) dessicated/shredded coconut
¼ cup (60 g/2 oz) raw sugar
Extra coconut for rolling

Place apricots in a bowl, pour over boiling water and leave to stand for 5 minutes. Drain well and pat dry with kitchen paper. Place apricots in a blender with coconut and sugar and process for 1 minute or until apricots are very finely chopped. Do not overprocess or the mixture will become too sticky. Add the sesame seeds and process until ingredients are well combined. Scoop out heaped teaspoons of the mixture and roll into balls. Roll in extra coconut until apricot balls are well coated. Chill in the refrigerator for a few hours or until firm.

HONEY JOYS

90 g/3 oz milk free margarine
1 tablespoon honey
⅓ cup sugar
4 cups cornflakes

Heat margarine, sugar and honey until mixture is frothy. Add cornflakes and mix well. Spoon into paper patty cases and bake in a slow oven for 10 minutes. Makes approximately 24.

TAHINI BISCUITS

185 g/16 oz tahini (sesame paste)
½ cup (150 ml/5 fl oz) honey
1½ cups (135 g/4½ oz) millet flakes or rice flakes
½ cup (60-90 g/2-3 oz) raisins or dates, or mixture
½ teaspoon cinnamon

Combine tahini and honey in bowl and gradually stir in nuts, etc and flakes mixed with cinnamon. Drop teaspoons onto greased biscuit tray and cook at 180°C/350°F/Gas 4 for about 10 minutes or until just beginning to brown.

PLAIN RICE BISCUITS (SWEET)

125 g/4 oz non dairy margarine
1 egg
salt
125 g/4 oz rice flour
125 g/4 oz sugar
Grated rind of ½ orange or lemon
125 g/4 oz cornflour/cornstarch

Cream margarine and sugar. Beat egg into above mixture. Add grated rind. Add sifted dry ingredients and mix well. Roll mixture into balls, place on a cold tray and flatten with fork. Bake at 190°C/375°F/Gas 5 for approximately 10 minutes.

CRACKLE SLICE

4 cups (100 g/3½ oz) rice bubbles
1 cup coconut
½ cup (60 g/2 oz) sunflower seeds
½ cup chopped cashews
2 tablespoon honey
2 tablespoon carob
½ cup currants
250 g/8 oz copha

Melt copha and cool slightly. Add to other ingredients. Press into flat container. Set in refrigerator, then cut into small squares.

WHITE CHRISTMAS (not cooked)

3½ cups rice bubbles
1½ cups coconut
1 cup (155 g/5 oz) mixed fruit
½ cup (90 g/3 oz) icing sugar/confectioner's sugar
1 cup dry soy milk or dry goat's milk
vanilla essence (pure)
250 g/8 oz copha

Melt copha and cool slightly. Add to all other ingredients. Press into flat container. Set in refrigerator then cut into small pieces.

APRICOT SLICE

1 tablespoon (15 g/½ oz) agar
1¼ cups water
2 tablespoons honey
⅓ cup oil or water
1 cup (125 g/4 oz) finely chopped dried apricots
1 cup sultanas/seedless raisins or chopped walnuts
½ cup sunflower seeds
1 cup rice flour
¾ cup (67 g/2¼ oz) rice flakes
½ cup (45 g/1½ oz) rice bran
⅓ teaspoon bicarbonate of soda/baking soda
1 teaspoon cream of tartar

Bring agar and water to the boil, simmer until the agar is partially dissolved. Add honey, oil, dried apricots, walnuts and sunflower seeds. Combine remaining ingredients together, mixing well. Stir in agar mixture. Spread over greased tray and bake in moderate oven 40-45 minutes.

CARROT CAKE

3 eggs, beaten
¼ cup honey
¾ cup oil
2 cups grated carrot
½ cup sunflower seeds, sultanas or walnuts, or mixture
170 g/5½ oz rice flour
2 teaspoons cinnamon
1 teaspoon bicarbonate of soda/baking soda
2 teaspoons cream of tartar
1 teaspoon vanilla

Lightly beat together eggs, honey and oil. Add carrot, nuts and vanilla. Mix together flour, bicarbonate of soda, cream of tartar and cinnamon and add to carrot mixture. Pour into greased and lined cake tin. Bake in moderate oven approximately 45 minutes.

ZUCCHINI CAKE

185 g/6 oz margarine (melted)
¾ cup (125 g/4 oz) black sugar
1½ cups grated zucchini/courgette
2 eggs, lightly beaten
1 cup (125 g/4 oz) fine polenta
½ cup potato flour
2 teaspoons (7 g/¼ oz) baking powder
⅓ cup (45 g/1½ oz) marzipan meal
½ cup (60 g/2 oz) slivered almonds
1 teaspoon cinnamon

Melt margarine in a medium to large saucepan. Remove from heat. Add sugar, zucchini, cinnamon, eggs. Sift flours and baking powder. Fold into mixture and add nuts and marzipan meal. Place in a lined and greased 20 cm/8″ spring form tin. Bake 1 hour at 180°C/350°F/Gas 4 for approximately 35 minutes.

COPHA CAKE

125 g/4 oz copha
¾ cup (185 g/6 oz) sugar
1 teaspoon vanilla (optional)
1 teaspoon baking powder
2 eggs
1 cup rice flour
1 cup cornflour/cornstarch
1 cup apple juice or soy milk

Have copha at room temperature. Beat copha and sugar until light and fluffy. Add eggs one at a time, beating well after each addition. Fold in sifted flour and baking powder alternately with liquid, add vanilla and beat mixture lightly until smooth. Spoon into shallow cake tin and bake in moderate oven (180°C/350°F/Gas 4 for approximately 35 minutes.

CORNFLOUR CAKE

250 g/8 oz milk free margarine
1 cup castor sugar
1¼ cups cornflour/cornstarch
4 large eggs
2 teaspoons baking powder

Beat together margarine and sugar, cornflour and eggs at medium speed in small bowl for 10 minutes. Time here is important. Add baking powder and beat one minute. Pour into greased 28 cm x 18 cm tin and bake in moderate oven (180°C/350°F/Gas 4) for 35 minutes. Can also be baked in 24 cm round tin for 50-60 minutes.

GINGER CAKE

60 g/2 oz non-dairy margarine
1 tablespoon (20 ml/⅔ fl oz) oil
2 cups (250 g/8 oz) plain flour/all purpose flour
2 eggs
2 teaspoons baking powder
2 tablespoons golden syrup, honey or treacle
¼ cup brown sugar (or 2 tablespoons (60 ml/2 fl oz) honey
1 teaspoon ground ginger
1 teaspoon mixed spice
pinch salt
1 teaspoon bicarb soda/baking soda
¾ cup water plus 2 tablespoons lactose free soy milk powder
½ cup buckwheat
½ cup cornflour starch
1 cup rice bran

Sift flour, spices and salt. Cream margarine and oil, sugar and syrup (or honey). Add eggs one at a time. Beat well. Add soy milk powder. Stir in other flours, alternating with water in which bicarbonate has been dissolved. Beat well. Mixture will look like thin batter mix. Cook for ¾ hour at 180°C/350°F/Gas 4.

PEANUT BUTTER AND BANANA BARS

1 egg, well beaten
⅓ cup peanut butter, or other nut butter
¼ cup molasses
½ cup brown rice flour or rice bran
½ cup (60 g/2 oz) walnuts or peanuts
1 ripe banana, chopped
¼ teaspoon cinnamon
¼ teaspoon sea salt

Preheat oven to 180°C/350°F/Gas 4. Combine all ingredients. Mix well. Turn into greased 20 cm/8″ pan and bake 15 minutes. Cut into bars while still warm.

NUT CAKE

500 gms/1 lb ground nuts, especially almonds and pecans
6 eggs, separated
2 tablespoons honey

Beat egg yolks and honey together. Stir in ground nuts. Fold in stiffly beaten egg whites. Bake in moderate oven about 40 minutes.

NUTAROONS

2 egg whites
¼ cup honey
¼ teaspoon almond essence
1 cup (90 g/3 oz) rice flakes
1 cup sunflower seeds
⅓ cup peanut butter (or other nut butter)
pinch salt

Beat egg whites until stiff. Combine honey and peanut butter. Add a small amount of egg white to peanut butter mixture to soften it, then fold in remainder of egg whites. Add other ingredients carefully. Drop small teaspoons onto a well greased baking tray. Bake for 10-15 minutes in a moderate oven, on the top shelf.

DATE CONFECTIONS

2 cups (315 g/10 oz) dates
½ cup (60 g/2 oz) pecans

Grind dates with pecans. Form into balls. Roll in coconut. Chill before serving.

Variations:
Use any other kind of nuts or seeds.

CAROB NUT CANDY

1 cup (120 g/4 oz) chopped walnuts (fine)
1 cup (90 g/3 oz) coconut
½ cup (60 g/2 oz) carob powder
½ cup (150 ml/5 fl oz) raw honey

Mix ingredients, kneading like dough. Add more coconut if necessary. Form into small bars. Chill before serving.

APRICOT CANDY

1 cup (60 g/2 oz) dried apricots
¼ cup (22 g/¾ fl oz) shredded coconut
orange juice

Soak apricots overnight. Drain. In blender, combine apricots with coconut and enough orange juice to make a firm dough. Form into balls. Roll with chopped almonds or coconut.

RAW FRUIT CAROB CANDY

2 cups (315 g/10 oz) pitted dates
1 cup (155 g/5 oz) seedless raisins
carob powder
½ cup (60 g/2 oz) chopped walnuts (optional)
½ cup (60 g/2 oz) sesame seeds

Grind together dates and raisins. Add walnuts. Add as much carob powder as mixture will hold. Roll into balls. Roll in roasted sesame seeds.

Variation:

Mix 1 cup sesame seeds (roasted and ground) with dates and raisins before adding carob.

SESAME CANDY

2 cups (250 g/8 oz) unhulled sesame seeds
1 tablespoon (2 ml/¾ fl oz) sesame oil (optional)
¼ cup (100 ml/¾ fl oz) honey
2 tablespoons (30 g/1 oz) tahini
Spices (optional)
1 teaspoon vanilla
¼ teaspoon cloves
½ teaspoon cinnamon
¼ teaspoon cardamon or coriander or nutmeg or mace
Mix all ingredients. Form into balls. Chill before serving.

SESAME TOFU

1 part sesame tahini
1 part honey (or to taste)
1 part kudzu arrowroot
5 parts water
Dissolve arrowroot in part of the water (cold). Mix remaining ingredients in thick bottomed saucepan. Heat gently to dissolve, then bring to the boil. Pour dissolved arrowroot in while beating with a wire fork or whisk. When thickened, cover, beat and cook slowly for about 20 minutes, while stirring and scraping the bottom of the pan. Pour into mould and let cool. Chill if desired. Spices can be used if desired.

FRESH FRUIT CAKE

1 cup oil (corn)
1 cup nut pieces
1 cup raisins
1 cup coconut
2 cups (185 g/6 oz) rolled oats
3 cups crushed fruit

½ *teaspoon salt*
1 *teaspoon vanilla*
2 *cups (250 g/8 oz) rice flour*
½ *cup (90 g/3 oz) potato starch*

Mix all ingredients to form soft slightly crumbling dough. Press into greased pans. Bake at 180°C/350°F/Gas 4 until golden. Cool and add date filling.

Date Filling

Simmer 250 g/8 oz dates with water to cover for 15 minutes. Mash into paste.

INTRODUCTION OF DAIRY AND GLUTEN PRODUCTS

After you have followed your particular dairy and wheat-free diet plan for four weeks you can start to test the different types of dairy products and wheat containing products. But remember that the majority of people need at least three months of total elimination of these products. You may react to cow's milk, for example, but not to goat's. You may find that milk or yogurt cause some adverse reaction but not hard cheese which has minimal amounts of lactose. Test them separately in very small quantities to start and watch for reactions. While testing, stay on the diet of the preceding month. When you test wheat make sure that you test a small quantity of a pure wheat product and not bread, which has yeast or malt in it. If you don't have severe reactions such as a rapid pulse elevation, increased blood glucose, a drop in post-meal salivary pH, changes in mood and behaviour, or other obvious physiological changes, or signs and symptoms previously mentioned, you can start to rotate the eliminated food back into the diet on a one week basis, then four days and finally every second day if you are not experiencing adverse reactions. Make sure you take your time when reducing the exposure frequency, and be careful of the slow increase in sensitivity which can take weeks to develop. In the final analysis you may find that you can tolerate hard cheese day one, goat's milk, day two, ricotta cheese and milk, day three, goat's yogurt, day four and so on. If this is too severe, alternate each day with nut milk, ie day one, goat's milk, day two, almond milk, day three, ricotta cheese, day four, cashew milk, day five, goat's yogurt, day six, soy milk, etc. You'll just have to try each scheme to find out which one is best for you.

Over the last few years interesting situations have arisen for some people at the time of re-challenge of suspected foods. On one occasion I received a visit from parents of two allergic children. They had decided to go on the same elimination diet as their children despite the fact that they had no observable signs of allergy themselves. After six weeks abstinence from various foods they suddenly experienced acute reactions from their first challenge of potatoes, bread, cheese, milk, sugar, onions, oats, corn and peanuts to name but a few. They were devastated to say the least. They could not understand what had happened. How could they have suddenly developed multiple allergies from just being on an elimination diet? The question they really wanted an answer to was, "Does this mean we will never be able to eat these foods again?" The answer was "no". They could eat all the foods again after the correct re-challenge and rotation procedure had been followed. This in fact happened.

From what I could gather the family had unmasked hidden food sensitivities to which they had become tolerant. They had also induced, nutritional deficiencies from not getting alternative dietary sources of vitamin A, riboflavin and calcium, when they eliminated dairy products from their diet. The parents were also under severe stress imposed by their particular elimination diet. Hence the elimination diet itself posed a serious nutritional and mental threat to the their health because of lack of guidance. In addition, at each food re-challenge the challenge dose was too high. For example, they challenged with dairy products for three successive days by having a glass of milk at each meal, a small container of yogurt daily, cream on desserts and about 2 x 50g cheese for snacks. In other words they really saturated their systems with dairy products after complete abstinence. This is like giving a dehydrated man in the desert a bucket of water to drink. Such reactions may, in some individuals, be no more than overwhelmed physiological responses due to a nutritionally and emotionally stressed body. These then combine with acute reactions from the unmasking of hidden cyclic allergies. With both children suffering from allergies there is a high possibility that one or both parents also had allergies, but had successfully adapted themselves to the stress of the allergens.

Most people can take 10 grams of sugar without displaying any symptoms of rebound hypoglycaemia. However the stress of not eating for 12 hours, plus a 75 gram glucose load which starts the glucose tolerance test are enough in themselves to cause severe hypoglycaemic symptoms.

In the case of the parents the elimination diet should have been nutritionally balanced and the eliminated foods recommenced in smaller quantities, such as a teaspoon of yogurt or a mouthful of milk on the first day while slowly increasing the quantity one week later, and then rotating the food into the diet at intervals of 4-7 days. Many food reactions at re-challenge can be eliminated simply by reducing the quantity of the reintroduced food and rotating it into the diet rather than presenting the food each day for three or four days. In this way the person with multiple cyclic food sensitivities can eat most foods without increasing their susceptibility to chronic disease at some future time, because the small quantity and wide spacing of the foods in the diet allows the body to adequately handle the reactive food.

Many books indicate that the quantity of the food is unimportant with cyclic allergies and the frequency of exposure is the all important factor. This is not so. If strict vegans eat a piece of steak or other animal protein after years of vegetarian food they will frequently become quite ill with nausea, vomiting, diarrhoea, etc. This is not a food allergy. This is the response of a body not used to handling meat proteins, especially in large quantities. The specific hormones in the body responsible for sensing food type vary with the composition of the diet. So does the ratio of protein digesting enzymes to carbohydrate digesting enzymes. The body's ratio of minerals, vitamins, amino acids and fatty acids is entirely dependent on the particular dietary balance of foods, and is reflected in differences in specific ratios of hormones, neurotransmitters, enzymes, etc, together with changes in physiological and biochemical processes. Sudden changes in the food composition of the diet can cause compensatory changes in the body's homeostatic mechanisms and physiological processes which may give rise to changes in heart rate, salivary pH, bowel movement frequency and composition and perhaps other symptoms indicative of physiological change – but these still do not constitute an allergic response. Emotional, mental and other lifestyle stresses can also be contributing to such internal body changes.

CHAPTER 8

NUTRITIONAL
INTERVENTION

NUTRITIONAL CONSIDERATIONS

Whenever staple foods are withdrawn completely from a diet or their frequency of consumption reduced severely there is always the possibility that nutritional deficiencies can arise.

Dairy products are perhaps our major source of riboflavin (vitamin B2) and calcium. It is therefore imperative that we substitute alternative foods containing these nutrients when we withdraw milk products from the diet. The potential for riboflavin deficiency is quite high when a pyridoxine (vitamin B6) supplement is administered together with a dairy-free diet. This is because vitamin B6 uses up vitamin B2 in the course of its biological reactions. Readily observable signs and symptoms such as sore, gritty, burning, light sensitive eyes, sore purplish tongue, cracked lips, hair loss and eczema are rapidly reversed by administering vitamin B2. We must be aware of such possibilities because we can quite easily mistake deficiency signs for actual manifestations of allergic reactions. In addition, when the body's nutritional status is seriously compromised by specific nutrient deficiencies, we are more prone to allergic reactions, and, in fact, such deficiencies may be a major factor in the aetiology of the allergic condition in the first place. Dr Lloyd Stills[46] demonstrated several years ago that about 15 per cent of children referred to him with chronic recurrent diarrhoea showed failure to thrive due to inadequate energy intake while on a strict elimination diet. Weight losses were rectified when the children resumed a normal diet.

Vegetarians with food intolerances are especially at risk if they can not tolerate eggs or dairy products, and special consideration has to be given to their food sources of essential amino acids, vitamin B12, riboflavin, and calcium. It is not uncommon for such people to slowly develop sensitivities to legumes, grains, seeds and nuts which are their major source of protein unless the foods are adequately rotated, while also keeping an eye on the food combinations which will supply all the amino acids at the same meal. It is no use obtaining the essential amino acids, isoleucine and lysine (predominantly in legumes) for lunch and tryptophan and the high sulphur containing amino acids (predominantly in grains, nuts and seeds) for dinner. The body must have all the essential amino acids together at a single meal.

Hence, the overall nutritional content on an elimination/rotation diet must be carefully considered. Alternative foods sources of riboflavin must be taken from soybeans, turnip greens, broccoli, mustard greens, asparagus, spinach, watercress, Brussels sprouts, cauliflower, squash (marrow) and some other vegetables. For meat eaters another good source is offal, for example liver. Some of the best alternative calcium sources to milk products are sesame seeds, tahini (ground hulled sesame seeds) almonds, adzuki beans, lima beans, soybeans, mustard greens, watercress, broccoli and cabbage. The best vegetable source of vitamin B12 is possibly the blue green algae called spirulina. Researchers from the University of Wisconsin[47] advise vitamin B12 supplementation for vegans or alternatively 1-3 grams/day of spirulina. Comfrey is not a good source because of the small quantity of vitamin B12 available and the possibility of ingesting carcinogens present in comfrey root.

If there is any doubt at all about the nutritional adequacy of the diet, take a wide spectrum vitamin and mineral supplement guaranteed by the manufacturers to be free of common allergenic excipients.

Another important consideration in designing a balanced diet is the fibre content of the foods. Since Burkitt[48] popularised the high fibre diet by associating lower fibre diets with a high incidence of colon cancer, diverticulitis, heart disease, diabetes and gall bladder problems (to name but a few) there has been a heavy and understandable emphasis on increasing the fibre content in the diet. While the most popular approach has been to add wheat bran to everything, this is possibly not the best approach, not only because of its wheat origin, but also because guar and other fibre components associated with legumes and vegetables may, in fact, prove to be superior fibre sources. Women on vegetarian diets have been shown to have lower incidences of breast cancer, possibly because of a class of substances called lignans derived from vegetables which are converted in the body to anti-cancer and anti-oestrogen substances called enterolactone, enterodial and equol.[49] Vegetarian-style diets also favourably alter oestrogen metabolism in women to further reduce the incidence of breast cancer.[50] Adequate fibre levels can be maintained during the rotation diets by effectively using whole corn, lentils, beans, peas, rice, sprouts, seeds, nuts and a great variety of vegetables. One fibre component called pectin actually activates the carbohydrate digesting enzyme in the pancreas called alpha-amylase, hence giving better digestion of carbohydrates. So the fibre content of the diet not only supplies roughage, it changes hormone levels and enzyme activities, and regulates the flow of digestive fluids, all of which may play an important role in minimising food intolerances.

THE USE OF NUTRITION SUPPLEMENTS

If used correctly and as a support, nutrition supplements can play a vital secondary role in optimising the biochemical reactions in the body, facilitating hormone and neuro-transmitter production, enhancing the host-defence mechanism by strengthening the immune system and supporting the digestive process. Nutritional support can act as a catalyst for quickly re-establishing the normal homeostatic mechanisms of the body which have been put out of balance. The key points to remember when using nutrition supplements is that they must be free of possible allergenic excipients such as corn, wheat, dairy products, yeast, soy, chemicals, sugar, artifical colouring and flavouring. The supplements themselves may still need to be rotated in the same manner as foods. Allergic reactions may arise from supplements such as pork derived pancreatin, soy-derived amino acids or lecithin, the wheat germ oil present in vitamin E capsules and so on. So read the labels carefully or ring the manufacturer if not sure.

Malabsorption frequently accompanies food intolerances. At such times the use of vegetable enzymes, pepsin and pancreatin can assist in the proper digestion of food and also help to digest potential offending food proteins which may be causing irritation of the gastro-intestinal tract, or which may even be absorbed systemically where they can act as irritants on the central nervous system (exorphins), cause inflammation of the joints as in arthritis, or may be the cause of skin reactions such as eczema or psoriasis, or inflammatory reactions in the lung such as asthma.

Many potential allergenic food reactions involving almost any part of the body can be controlled effectively with the use of digestive enzyme supplements combined with a rotation diet. The body may become quite acidic after the ingestion of an allergenic food. Some people can reduce this acidity by taking ½ teaspoon of a specific bicarbonate preparation (two parts sodium bicarbonate and one part potassium bicarbonate) about ½ to one hour after the meal together with pancreatic enzyme supplements. Bicarbonate activates these enzymes, and hence, aids in protein digestion, helps reduce the metabolic acidosis accompanying the food reaction and can actually act as an antidote for many food reactions if one heaped teaspoon is taken 30 minutes after the food and with several glasses of water. Bicarbonate must not be taken together with ascorbic acid and should not be used continually.

Another aid to malabsorption is the use of mixed amino acid supplements (hydrolysed or predigested protein). If fat digestion is a problem the micellised form of vitamins A and E have been shown to be highly effective, even in cases of cystic fibrosis and pancreatitis where the normal fat soluble vitamins are not absorbed.

Recent research has highlighted the important role of several fatty acids in the treatment of disorders arising from food intolerances such as eczema and asthma. These fatty acids are called gamma-linolenic acid, which is found in evening primrose oil, and eicosapent-aenoic acid (EPA), which is present in large amounts in oils derived from fatty cold water fish such as salmon, sardines and herring. These important fatty acids are vital for the formation of substances in the body called prostaglandins which control inflammatory reactions producing redness, swelling, oedema and pain, and also other aspects of the immune system.

The supplements I have found to be of greatest value for the treatment of disorders related to food intolerance are: pyridoxine (vitamin B6); pantothenic acid (vitamin B5); folic acid, vitamin B12, vitamin A, vitamin C, vitamin E, zinc, magnesium, iron, manganese, and copper.

The justification for this selection is mainly based on scientific reports plus my own clinical experience, but several key areas of metabolism may be shown to depend on many of these micronutrients. Vitamins B5 and B6, for example, are vital for the formation of cortisone and other steroids as well as the production and control of an important regulating molecule in the pituitary gland called ACTH (adrenocorticotrophic hormone). Vitamin B6 also controls amino acid metabolism which is frequently disordered during maladaptive food reactions, and has also proved to be an effective agent for reducing fluid (oedema). The combination of zinc, magnesium, vitamin B6, vitamin C and vitamin E are the major catalysts for the production of prostaglandins from fatty acids as described previously.

Finally, each one of the seven vitamins and five minerals controls and directs the optimal functioning of our host defence mechanism. Deficiences of any of these micronutrients may seriously reduce the functioning of our immune system, according to a 1981 workshop sponsored by the Department of Food and Nutrition and its Nutrition Advisory Group of the American Medical Association.[51] The workshop showed that the individuals may need increased amounts of certain vitamins and minerals when malnutrition results from medical illness. Impaired immunocompetence can lead to increased respiratory, skin and intestinal complaints, a situation very reminiscent of food intolerance. The vitamins shown by the workshop to have the most important immunological effects were the water soluble vitamins pyridoxine (vitamin B6), pantothenic acid (vitamin B5) and ascorbic acid (vitamin C), as well as the fat soluble vitamins A and E. The minerals with the most well defined role were iron and zinc.‡

‡ *The evidence of important immunological roles for these vitamins and minerals uncovered by this workshop and also by other investigators is worth summarising.*[52, 53, 54, 55]

PYRIDOXINE (VITAMIN B6)

Pyridoxine deficiency has been the most extensively studied B vitamin deficiency condition in the field of immunology. It interferes with the normal synthesis of protein and DNA in lymphocyte proliferation when stimulated by antigens. Low blood levels of lymphocytes is a common finding in most species tested. In both people and animals experimental vitamin B6 deficiency has led to a poor antibody response to either primary or booster immunizations. This is most probably due to a reduction in quantity of specific antibodies as well as defects in the antibodies that are produced. Hence, the importance of ensuring high vitamin status, especially in children before immunisation programs. It is possible that some of the rare side effects associated with mass immunisation programs are related to low vitamin status.

When combined vitamin B6 and B5 deficiency occurs together, the immunological deficit is even more striking. In one study of healthy human volunteers made B5 and B6 deficient, antibody response to tetanus toxoid and typhoid antigens was almost completely inhibited. An induced puridoxine deficiency leads to a 50 per cent reduction in peripheral blood lymphocyte count, a marked reduction in thoracic duct (a major storage depot of lymphocytes) lymphocytes from 90 million cells/ml to approximately 5 million. There was also a massive reduction and change in distribution of T and B cells (the two major types of lymphocytes) from the thoracid duct lymph. The remaining T cells were not only markedly depleted, but also functionally impaired.

In 1965 an analysis of patients with common disorders at a New Jersey hospital revealed 26 per cent with pyridoxine deficiency.

PANTOTHENIC ACID (VITAMIN B5)

Pantothenic acid deficiency in man and animals reduces antibody responses to immunisation by inhibiting the stimulation of antibody producing cells, and the subsequent production of immunoglobulins by the B-cells. This effect, as previously stated, is further exacerbated by a combined deficiency of vitamins B5 and B6. When rats deprived of pantothenic acid were challenged with sheep antigens (foreign protein derived from sheep) there was a depressed antibody response. Primary antibody-forming cells from the spleen were reduced from 20 per million spleen cells to 8 per million. A rebound improvement occurred (318 antibody-forming cells per million) when vitamin B5 deficient rats were given pantothenic acid just before immunisation.

ASCORBIC ACID (VITAMIN C)

When the healthy human volunteers were given one gram ascorbic acid each day over a 10-week period, their serum immunoglobulin A and M levels were significantly increased, compared to another group who received no vitamin C supplements. A deficiency in vitamin C in guinea pigs caused impaired graft rejection, with skin grafts surviving 2½ times longer than controls. Other studies with guinea pigs suggest that the immune inhibitory effect of vitamin C deficiency is due to the reduced production or activity of various peptide hormones found in the thymus gland. There is a linear increase in the weight of lymph nodes and spleen directly proportional to ascorbic acid intake. Ascorbate (vitamin C) concentrations 10-50 times that of normal plasma levels have been observed to increase random mobility of leukocytes and hence their effectiveness.

Vitamin C has been shown to increase the rate at which lymphocyte DNA and protein are synthesised. The effects of increasing weekly doses of ascorbate on certain immune functions in normal volunteers was reported in 1980 in the American Journal of Clinical Nutrition. Supplementary vitamin C increased the rate of division of B-lymphocytes into antibody producing cells by up to three times when subjects were given up to 3,000 mg vitamin C. It is interesting to note that when vitamin C is given with aspirin the leukocyte vitamin C level is significantly higher than resting levels.

VITAMIN A

A deficiency of vitamin A in animals can lead to an increased frequency and severity of bacterial, viral and protozoan infections or a depletion of T-lymphocytic response to antigens. Atrophy of the thymus gland (where T-lymphocytes are matured) has occurred when vitamin A deficiency is combined with protein-calorie malnutrition. Supplementation with vitamin A helps to maintain the integrity of epithelial and mucosal surfaces and their secretions. It improves resistance to bacterial and fungal infections, antibody response and cell mediated immunity (such as an accelerated graft rejection if given from five days before to 10 days after grafting). When vitamin A was added to human peripheral blood lymphoctyes, increased lymphocyte proliferative response was achieved with very small amounts of vitamin A and was dose dependent.

VITAMIN E

Vitamin E deficiency in animals causes a general reduction in host resistance, delayed skin hypersensitivity reactions, reduced proliferative response of lymphocytes to antigens and a depressed response of immunoglobulins to antigens. In doses up to 10 times greater than the minimum daily allowance, vitamin E has been shown to enhance both antibody reactions to animal vaccines and delayed skin hypersensitivity reactions. It can also accelerate the clearance of cellular debris, offer greater host resistance and ability to survive experimental infections, although one report stated that megadoses of vitamin E given to healthy volunteers inhibited multiple immune functions.

IRON

Iron is required for the maintenance of lymphoid tissue and iron deficiency can cause atrophy of such tissues with impaired lymphocyte responsiveness to foreign agents. In animals, antibody production decreases with as little as a 10 per cent decrease in iron. Frequently investigators' findings are contradictory, possibly because of coexisting nutrient deficiences, infection or protein calorie malnutrition in experimental subjects. Various studies have shown a higher prevalence of acute and chronic infections in iron-deficiency anaemia patients, but other workers have demonstrated fewer infections in this type of anameia. In 20 children with iron-deficient anaemia, T-cell levels were significantly depressed in 49 per cent compared with 63 per cent in the control group.

ZINC

Zinc is most certainly the leader of the team of minerals involved in maintaining immunocompetence. A deficiency of zinc is associated with: atrophy of lymphoid tissues; impaired antibody response; impaired cell-mediated immunity with depressed T-cell activity and a lack of delayed cutaneous hypersensitivity reactions and skin graft rejections; thymic atrophy and suppression of thymic hormone activity.

Immune functions can be restored, however, in zinc deficient patients upon zinc repletion.

Evidence is rapidly accumulating which gives testimony for the active role of the immune system in most of the chronic degenerative disorders currently found in our Western society. Asthma, eczema, gastrointestinal complaints and autoimmune disorders such as multiple sclerosis, rheumatoid arthritis, scleroderma, lupus erythematosus and other collagen diseases are all associated with either underactivity, overactivity or imbalance in the immune system. Supplementation with the key immunological micronutrients is just another aid which may help to restore balance to a system working under severe stress. The use of freeze dried thymus gland supplements may also be considered where autoimmune disorders are related to food sensitivities. Hormones from the thymus gland may be helpful in stabilising and controlling the production of T-lymphocytes and the elaboration of antibodies by the B-lymphocytes.

If you are thinking of using nutritional supplements during the treatment of food intolerances it is recommended that you see a nutritionally oriented health professional first.

CHAPTER 9

COPING

WITH

CHILDREN

PREGNANCY AND INFANT FEEDING

If you are thinking of becoming pregnant you should start to maximise your exercise program, remove all junk foods from your diet, eliminate as many stress factors from your environment as you can identify, including cigarettes and alcohol. Under no circumstances go on a fast if there is any likelihood that you are pregnant as this may affect foetal development. If you have any idea that you may have food intolerances start to rotate your foods.

Rotate all foods including wheat and dairy products unless you have certain fixed allergies in which case you completely remove the offending foods during the entire period of your pregnancy and lactation. You can well do without physiological stressors during the period of gestation. It may be wise, however, to include foods on a rotation basis to which you have mild reactions if continually exposed to such a food. Animal studies have suggested that complete abstinence from a substance such as wheat during pregnancy resulted in a greater sensitivity to wheat in the offspring compared to offspring which had some exposure to wheat in utero. Presumably by rotating such a food in the diet during pregnancy the foetus is exposed periodically, but not continually to potential food antigens and develops a better mechanism for coping with them as a neonate.

It is equally important for the mother to rotate her foods (if she has food intolerances) during the period of lactation. This is because allergenic food components which have not been adequately processed by the mother can be transferred to the child via the mother's breast milk. This may result in allergic symptoms such as diarrhoea, colic, running nose, wheezing or even eczema before the child has been weaned.

A report in the Journal of Clinical Allergy in 1980 gives further evidence for this potential to transfer allergens from mother to child. The reports noted two fully breast fed infants who developed signs of food allergy. The allergens were from cow's milk and/or egg and appeared to be transferred via the mother's breast milk after the mother had eaten one of the reactive foods. Breast milk sampled one hour after one of the mothers had ingested egg produced a positive skin test reaction in her infant. When milk was sampled from another nursing mother one hour after she had eaten egg, this mother's milk did not produce a positive skin reaction in the same infant. These results indicate that food allergens may be transmitted to an infant via the breast milk of the mother, though not necessarily from the breast milk of a surrogate mother. Obviously in this case the surrogate mother also ate the egg but did not transfer any allergenic component of the egg through the breast milk.

While giving due attention to these ideas it still cannot be overemphasised that infants should be breast fed for a minimum of six months and preferably 12 months. The virtues of breast feeding over cow's milk and formulas have been adequately covered elsewhere,[57] but it should be noted that the practice of formula feeding has some additional disadvantages which are not always highlighted. Quite apart from the allergenicity of soy or cow's milk and the differences in protein content, vitamins, fatty acids and trace elements, the formulas lack some very important biological molecules called enzymes.

The neonate and infant during the first six months has a suboptimal level of digestive enzymes, and, in fact, the major carbohydrate digesting enzymes in the infant's pancreas in some cases, may not be fully functional until about 6-7 months of age. This alone is an important reason for withholding grains, legumes, and other starch-containing foods from the infant until at least six months of age. Even the protein and fat digesting enzymes of the infant do not operate optimally for several weeks post-partum. Human milk, however, is loaded with digestive enzymes that help the digestion of the milk.[58] This digestive support within breast milk may be more important than we think and may actually contribute to the digestion of potential allergenic proteins within the mother's milk once the milk reaches the infant's gastrointestinal tract. Such support is not forthcoming from soy-based milk or even cow's milk which has a different spectrum of enzymes and has lost enzyme activity through pasturisation.

ROTATION OF FORMULAS

If breast feeding is completely out of the question for any reason, try rotation of formulas so that the baby is not exposed to the same foreign proteins every four hours, even if the rotation only includes goat's milk and soy milk (or if absolutely necessary cow's milk). Rotation will reduce the tendency towards intolerance and will also maximise nutrition, as many micronutrients missing in one formula may be found in another or an incorrect mineral ratio may tend to normalise by extending the nutrient source. This procedure will of course depend upon the infant's acceptance of more than one formula. Under no circumstances should a woman feel guilty for not breast feeding or for introducing various suspect foods too soon into an infant's diet. Some women suffer in this way after they discover that they may have been able to prevent many of their children's allergenic manifestations if they had 'only known what to do' during pregnancy and the post-natal period. These feelings only serve to increase the stress load of the mother and are really quite counter-productive. With allergies you can *never* be absolutely sure of *any* correct procedure.

INTRODUCTION OF SOLIDS (6-12 MONTHS)

Try starting with well cooked, sieved or blended pumpkin, potato, carrot, rice-cream, lamb, fish, turkey, chicken, pear, banana, beetroot, sago, brains, vegetable soups, tofu, thinned avocado and pawpaw, choko, spinach, zucchini and other bland vegetables. For juices try fresh diluted vegetables juices, strained cashew and almond milks, goat's milk, soy milk, diluted fruit juices.

As new foods are introduced into the diet always be on the look out for changes in bowel movements (either frequency or consistency), stomach aches, increased wind, increased waking, pot belly, eczema, wheezing, ear, nose and throat problems. Such observations can herald the first signs of food intolerances. You need to watch for them, however, as these changes can quite easily go unobserved or be taken for granted or put down to teething problems or an inner feeling that all babies have colic and other minor problems so why worry.

In view of the frequency with which children show intolerances to cow's milk, wheat products and eggs it is preferable to postpone the introduction of these foods for the first six months and if possible for the first 12 months. When introducing any new food, however, start with a very small amount. Several drops or ½ teaspoon is adequate and slowly increase the quantity while rotating at approximately four-day intervals.

TRIPLE ANTIGEN

Children can sometimes react adversely to innoculations for diptheria, whooping cough or tetanus and also to the oral solution for protection against polio. The best way to minimise these reactions is to:

• Make sure the child has no fever, infections or any form of illness at the time of innoculation.

• One week before, through to one week after innoculation, take a multivitamin and mineral formula together with 1-2 grams each day of vitamin C. These vitamins and minerals will maximise the immune response to the vaccines (ie optimise function of thymus gland and production of lymphocytes and antibodies, and activity of other white blood cells). The specific vitamins and minerals which are most important for a correct functioning immune system are vitamins B5, B6, B12, C, E, A, folate, zinc, iron, manganese, copper and magnesium. In this way you make sure of optimising the body's antibody response to the innoculation antigen and also help reduce side effects from the vaccines as well as any possible allergic reactions to other components in the injections.

• Ask your doctor to separate the vaccines of the triple antigen and administer them over a period of several months (especially the one for whooping cough). This reduces the antigenic load at any one time by ⅓. This procedure is highly recommended for children with pre-existing allergies and who already have a load placed on their immune system. There has been a suggestion of possible allergic reactions to the materials used for producing the vaccines.

GETTING CHILDREN TO EAT THE NEW FOODS

Compliance with adults is hard enough. For children it can sometimes seem impossible. The dietary restrictions are frequently too hard to follow and the strain on the entire family becomes obvious. For example, lack of compliance may arise because the infant is allowed to become a fussy eater and tends to narrow the range of foods down to just a few allergenic foods which the infant craves and subsequently becomes addicted to. Some children will only eat three or four different foods. Mothers often find it impossible to make their children eat the recommended foods until all of the suspected foods have been removed from the household. The new foods may be slowly introduced by either mixing with a food the child likes (such as adding rice, carrot, pumpkin and peas to hamburgers and rissoles, or adding fruit and nuts to blended drinks such as soy milk and cashew milk). The other way is to make your own bread out of corn, rice, rye, potato flour, etc in place of wheat flour. Similarly, make your own pie crusts with your own filling. In other words, the children can still eat their favourite foods if you alter the composition of the foods. The chocolate milkshake suddenly becomes blended almonds, banana and carob; lemonade becomes mineral water with real lemon and honey added and so on. Try grating pumpkin into coleslaw or making pumpkin chips instead of potato chips. This kind of lateral thinking can often produce the desired effect, despite undesirable socially induced food preferences in the child.

Another good way to increase the variety of foods in the diet is to get the child involved with food preparation. This can begin with choosing vegetables or fruit in the shop and later helping with their preparation, especially if the food is to be cooked.

Sometimes the actual shape or design of the new food can be changed in some way to make the food more appealing. For example, apples and pears can be cored and cut horizontally to form donut shapes. A banana can be sliced lengthways into a boat shape with a thin slice of apple on a toothpick for the sail. You can make faces in vegetables such as tomatoes, by inserting two carrot slices for eyes and one for the mouth using a vegetable peeler for the carrots. Kids love to help in the preparation of such fun food, and, eventually, are more likely to try some. Try eating with chopsticks one night. Have a meat fondue where the kids can cook their own dinner at the table, or cook a Japanese sukiyaki which requires fresh ingredients to be cooked at the table. Try presenting foods on toothpicks or skewers. Let them serve themselves from a smorgasbord setting. This gets around the idea that you are forcing them to eat any specific foods. Many mothers tell me that the best way to introduce a new food into the diet is to make sure it is presented on the plate each night, but after the first night of coaxing the child, just forget about it and frequently within a week or so the child has started to eat the food. This illustrates the advantages of not *forcing* children to eat a specific food.

Expose children to as wide a variety of foods as possible. Try a new food each week and keep a positive attitude at the dinner table at all times. There are hundreds of foods to choose from, but we commonly make selections from no more than a few dozen foods. By giving a child a choice of foods you will often get them eating a greater variety. Cafeteria feeding experiments with children have shown that they frequently know what foods their body requires as long as their tastes have not been corrupted with too many concentrated flavours, sugar and salt excesses, and as long as you control the foods available (ie no allergenic foods according to a rotated schedule as they cannot eat the same food every day).

SCHOOL LUNCHES

School lunches are mainly a problem because conventional sandwiches cannot be used if the child is on a gluten-free diet. Social pressure limits any imaginative attempts by the mother to circumvent the problem. Other children are very prone to single out the boy or girl with the strange lunch box. However, a lot depends on the personality of the child. Supposing a little girl is an outward-going type. You may tell her to say to the other kids (when they are eating their sandwiches): 'Not sandwiches again – you've had them every day this week. Look what I've got today,' or 'don't you get tired of the same old sandwiches every day?' If, however, this type of approach will not work for your child there are a certain number of socially acceptable foods which you can try. These include: rissoles, meatballs, chicken legs, wheat-free cold sausages, cobs of corn, cold lamb chops or lamp shanks, pieces of fruit, nuts, dried fruit. Some children can rotate 100 per cent rye bread if they have a wheat sensitivity but not a gluten sensitivity. Other breads, biscuits or cake can be made from corn, rice, potato or soya flour. During the cold weather a soup in a vacuum flask can be enough in itself if it contains vegetables, gains, legumes or meat. Soups are frequently served from canteens, but check to see that they don't include canned soup which usually contains wheat flour. You may even go so far as to use the same paper cups for your soup that are actually used in the canteen, if this type of social conformity will help your child. Summer lunches such as salads can be kept cool by packing them with refrigerated ice packs.

For children who don't tend to eat lunch anyway because they would rather play, just give them fruit and let them have a substantial meal (ie in a crockpot or a salad) when they get home from school. They also need a substantial breakfast or you will have a little monster on your hands by 3 pm.

BIRTHDAY PARTIES

Try to eliminate all birthday parties during the first month of the diet program unless they are at your own home in circumstances where you are in control of the food. In this way you can still prepare delicious cakes, sweets, etc, which are dairy and wheat-free and also low in sugar (see recipes). You can, for example, make chocolate crackles using carob; gelato is a good dairy-free ice cream substitute, or you can make ice cream using cashew or almond milks. Ice blocks can be made from pure fruit juice. Pineapple boats and water melon balls can be a real hit with the kids.

After the first month the situation changes. Allergies are usually unmasked, and at this stage a good burst of rubbish food may be quite enlightening for both parents and child. At worst, the child's behaviour suddenly deteriorates, moods swing, tensions flare and often there is a sudden return of signs and symptoms such as running noses, wheezing, headaches, glue ear, stomach aches, diarrhoea, wakeful nights and bed wetting. Usually, however, these symptoms only persist for a few days as there is a slow reversion to the unmasked state again, this time at a much faster rate. So such an event can be quite informative. If no symptoms are observed it may indicate that some of the restricted foods can now be rotated back into the diet on a seven-day or four-day basis. The rotation frequency, however, is a highly individual thing and cannot be predicted.

SUPPLEMENTARY PROGRAMS FOR CHILDREN

Many of the children I have treated with learning difficulties, balance and co-ordination problems, minimal brain dysfunction and a wide variety of other inappropriate behaviour patterns, have responded very well to a combination of nutritional/dietary manipulation, together with a modified program of sensory intergrative therapy. This modified program is presently run in my area by a colleague,[59] who is an occupational therapist, and basically consists of specific stimulation of appropriate sensory systems in play form. Special equipment is designed to stimulate tactile, proprioceptive and vestibular systems in a variety of combinations, together with balance and co-ordinated use of two sides of the body. A simple motor planning program is then taught to show the child how to use his/her newly acquired skills. Body scheme activities include forward rolls, pencil rolls, backwards rolls, crab crawls, wheelbarrows, hand clapping involving cross-over patterns, skipping through a big rope in turn, stopping and starting with hopping and skipping and other variables often following the children's suggestions.

Sensory integrative therapy helps children who have difficulties conceiving, organising and carrying out a sequence of unfamiliar actions or performing new tasks. For example, learning to ride a dinky or bike requires holding the steering wheel with two hands, turning the wheel, operating the pedals, directing the vehicle from A to B. The new tasks initially require the cortex or thinking part of the brain to learn the activities which then quickly become automated. Then the child can perform the task effortlessly without having to think about it. An inability to learn and integrate such demands may lead to an inability to automate such activities, and hence great efforts and inappropriate responses result.

A similar situation applies if a child cannot learn to write words without thinking or cannot walk up steps without looking at their feet. Such problems with automating newly acquired/skills involving fine or gross motor movements lead to co-ordination and balance problems in the child. It may become clumsy, have great difficulty learning to write or play the piano. This subsequently leads to the child having a poor self image, lack of confidence and self control, and, if highly intelligent, the tendency to show extremely frustrated reactive behaviour.

Many social, emotional and physical problems in some children may be traced back to such poorly functioning pre-requisites of sensory input and the resultant attempts to compensate for such inadequacies.

REFERENCES

1. Kraehenbuhl, JP & Campiche, WA *J. Cell. Biol.* 42, 345-365 (1969)
2. Udall, JN et.al. *Pediatr. Res.* 15, 241-249 (1981)
3. Matthew, DJ et.al. *Lancet* I, 321-324 (1977)
4. Jackson, PG et.al. *Lancet* I, 1285-1286 (1981)
5. Manuel, PD et.al. *Lancet* II, 1365-1366 (1980)
6. Hosking, et.al. *Brit. Med. J.* 283, 693-696 (1981)
7. Heiner, DC, *N. Eng. J. Med.* 304, No 1, 55 (1981)
8. Lecks, HI, *JAMA* 244, No 14, 1560 (1980)
9. Korenblat, RE et.al. *J. Allergy* 41, 226-235 (1968)
10. Park, A & Hughes, G, *Brit. Med. J.* 282, 2027-2029 (1981)
11. Bowerman, WM, *J. Ortho. Psych.* 9, No 4, 263-267 (1980)
12. Swain, A & Unsworth, DJ, *J. Roy. Soc Med.* 74, 458-459 (1981)
13. Hemmings, G (Ed.) *The Biochemistry of Schizophrenia & Addiction* p. 169-176 MTP Press (1980)
14. Dohen, FC & Grasberger, JC *Am.J. Psychiatry,* 130, 685 (1973)
15. Singh, MM & May SR, *Science* 191, 401 (1976)
16. Dohan, FC, *Adv. Biochem. Psychopharmacol.* 22, 535-548 (1980)
17. Dohan, FC, *N. Eng. J. Med.,* 302, No 22, 1262 (1980)
18. Dohan, FC, *Acta. Neurol.* (Napoli) 31, 195 (1976)
19. Dohan, FC, *Am.J.Clin.Nutr.* 18, 7 (1966)
20. Mascord I, *Brit. Med. J.* 1, 1351 (1978)
21. Radcliffe et al. *The Practitioner* 225, 1651-1654 (1981)
22. Monro, J et.al. *Lancet* II, 1-4 (1980)
23. Ogle KA & Bullock, JD, *Annals of Allergy* 44, 273-278 (1980)
24. Cavagni, C, *The Practitioner,* 225, 1657-1660 (1981)
25. Lake-Bakaa, G et.al., *Gut* 21, 580-586 (1980)
26. *Diet Crime and Delinquency* by Schauss, 13-14 Parker House (1981)
27. *The Role of Nightshade Plants in Arthritis,* presented to the International Academy of Preventive Medicine, St.Louis (1979)
28. Mandell, M & Conte, A, *J.Int.Acad.Prevent.Med* VII, No 2, 5-16 (1982)

29. Jenkins, DJ, *Am.J.Clin.Nutr.* 36, 1093-1101 (1982)
30. Crapo, PA et.al., *Am.J.Clin.Nutr.* 33, 1723-1728 (1980)
31. Bolton, RP et.al., *Am.J.Clin.Nutr.* 34, 211-217 (1981)
32. O'Dea, K. et.al., *Am.J.Clin.Nutr.* 34, 1991-1993 (1981)
33. Collier, G & O'Dea, K, *Am.J.Clin.Nutr.* 36, 10-14 (1982)
34. Krause, MV & Mahan, LK, *Food, Nutrition & Diet Therapy*, 6th Ed. p 500, WB Saunders Company (1979)
35. Yudkin, J, *Am.J.Clin.Nutr.* 34, 1453 (1981)
36. *Nutr. Metab.* 24, 182-188 (1980)
37. Reiser, et.al. *Am.J.Clin.Nutr.* 32, 1659 (1979)
38. Kamath, K & Hill, R, *Medical J.Aust.* 1,9, 387-389 (1982)
39. Philpott, WH & Kalita, DK, *Brain Allergies* p 115-125, Keats Publishing, Inc. (1980)
40. Golos, N & Golbitz, FG, *Coping with your Allergies,* Simon & Schuster (1979)
41. Randolph, TG & Moss, RW, *An Alternative Approach to Allergies* Lippincott & Crowell (1980)
42. McGovern, JJ, *Food & Chem. Toxicol.,* 20,4,491 (1982)
43. McGovern, JJ, et.al., *Int.J.Biosoc Res.* 4, (1) 40-42 (1983)
44. Coca, A, *The Pulse Test* ARCO Publ.Inc. (1979)
45. Randolph, TG, in *Clinical Ecology* Ed. L Dickey p 577-596, Charles C Thomas Publ. 1976
46. Lloyd-Stills, J, *J.Pediat.* 95, 10-13 (1979)
47. Dong, A & Scott, S. *Annals of Nutrition & Metabolism* 26, 209-216 (1982)
48. Burkitt, DP et.al. *JAMA* 229, 1068 (1974)
49. Adlercrentz, H et.al. *Lancet* II, 1295-1298 (1982)
50. Goldin, BR et.al. *N.Eng.J. Med.* 307, 1542-1547 (1982)
51. Nutrition Advisory Group of the AMA – *JAMA* 245, 53-58 (1981)
52. Dreizen, S. Internat. *J. Vit. Nutr. Res.* 49, 120-128 (1979)
53. Gross, RL & Newberne, PM, *Physiological Reviews* 60, No 1, 188-302 (1980)
54. Beisel, WR, *Am.J.Clin.Nutr.* 35, (Supplement) No. 2, February 1892)
55. Cunningham-Rundles, S., *Am.J.Clin.Nutr.* 35, 1202-1210 (1982)
56. *Journal of Clinical Allergy* 10, 133-136 (1980)
57. Blanc, B. *Wld.Rev.Nutr.Diet* 36, 1-89 (Karger, Basle 1981)
59. Mrs Marj Allnut
60. Truss, C, *J.Orthomulecular Psychiatry* 9, No 4, 287-301 (1980)
61. Egger, J et.al., *Lancet* II, 865-868 (1983)

GLOSSARY

Addison's disease   a deficiency in the secretion of adrenal gland hormones

allergen   any substance that causes allergic manifestations (usually a protein)

allergenic   causing an allergic reaction

antibodies   special proteins made by the body to fight foreign agents (usually proteins called antigens)

antigens   a substance that induces the formation of an antibody

auto-immune disorders   diseases where the body turns the immunological process against itself

arrowroot   used as a thickener

agar   used to thicken or make jelly/gelatin

beetroot/beet

bicarbonate of soda   also known as baking soda

capsicum   red or green pepper

calamari   cooked squid

challenges   re-exposure to possible allergenic food

chickory   also known as witloof, French or Belgian endive

chips   also known as French fries

corn   maize

double-blind   neither investigators nor patients know which is the active substance

eggplant   aubergine

fetta cheese   sheep's cheese (but some Australian fetta is made with cow's milk)

fatty acids   constituent molecules of oils or fat

filbert   substitute hazelnut

gelatin   jelly

garam marsala   mixture of Asian spices

glucometer   a device for measuring blood sugar levels

glucose tolerance test   measurement of glucose tolerance

hijiki   seaweed

hypopituitarism   diminished secretion of pituitary gland

immune complexes   a combination of antigen and antibody

insulinoma   a tumor of the insulin secreting cells of the pancreas

immunoglobulins   proteins which are capable of acting as antibodies

jelly   Australia and UK, gelatin, USA

kiwi fruit   Chinese gooseberry. A green fruit with a brown furry skin. Other varieties of gooseberry may be substituted.

kudzu   a thickening agent like arrowroot

lettuce   of the many lettuce varieties available, the recipes generally refer to iceberg — USA, Webb's wonder — UK, common lettuce — Australia. However other varieties may be used where available.

mignonette lettuce   round/cabbage lettuce or Boston bibb lettuce

marrow   squash

miso   concentrated soy paste

nephropathy   a general term for diseases of the kidney

okra   gumbo in the UK, ladies' fingers in the USA

paw paw   papaya

placebo   an inactive substance thought by the patient to be active

plain flour   all purpose flour

platelets   specialized white blood cells

psoriasis   a skin disease causing red scaly patches.

runner beans   string beans, green beans

rockmelon   cantaloupe

retinopathy   any disorder of the retina

sultanas   seedless raisins

sweet potato   yam

swede   rutabaga

taboulie   Lebanese green salad

tamari   naturally fermented soy sauce

tahini   sesame seed paste

vanilla   vanilla essence

zucchini   courgettes

RECIPES
INDEX

DESSERTS

BAKED FOODS & SNACKS

ALPHABETICAL INDEX

salicylates *17, 52*
saliva pH test *59*
schizophrenia *11, 17-21*
scleroderma *208*
school lunches *214*
senses *46-48*
sensory integrative therapy *216*
skim milk *20*
snack recipes *183*
somnolence *28*
soup recipes *113*
spirulina *202*
sprays *51*
starches *39*
starters (recipes) *134*
stress *48-50*
stressors *27-30, 41, 42*
stress reduction *43*
sucrose *39*
sugar *38-41*
supplements *203*
synovitis *20*

T

tetanus *212*
thymus gland *208*
thymus gland supplements *208*
thoughts *48*
triglycerides *39*
triple antigen *212*

U
unmasking *28, 30, 197*
uric acid *39*

V

vegetable dishes *128*
vegetable enzymes *204*
vitamin A *205*
vitamin B2 (riboflavin) *201*
vitamin B5 (pantothenic acid) *205, 206*
vitamin B6 (pyridoxine) *201, 205, 206*
vitamin B12 *202*
vitamin C *58, 205, 206*
vitamin E *203, 205, 207*
vomiting *28*

W

waffle recipes *104*
water miscible vitamins *205*
wheat *12, 23, 29, 34, 61, 213*
wheat bran *203*
wheat germ oil *203*
wheat substitutes *102*
whey *24*
whooping cough *212*
withdrawal symptoms *28*

X, Y, Z

yeast *13, 61*
yogurt *35, 64*
zinc *205, 208*